Survival of the
Thinnest

Survival of the
Thinnest

How to Use Your Genetic Script
to Stay Thin Without Dieting

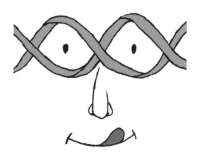

David Hariton

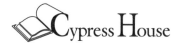

Cypress House

Survival of the Thinnest
How to Use Your Genetic Script to Stay Thin Without Dieting
Copyright © 2004 by David Hariton.
www.survivalofthethinnest.com

Cypress House
155 Cypress Street
Fort Bragg, California 95437
800-773-7782   Fax: 707-964-7531

http:\\www.cypresshouse.com

Book production by Cypress House

Cover and interior illlustrations by Scott Menchin

Book design by Michael Brechner

Cataloging-in Publication Data

Hariton, David P.
  Survival of the thinnest : how to use your genetic script to stay thin without dieting / David P. Hariton. -- 1st ed. -- Fort Bragg, CA : Cypress House, 2003.
   p. ; cm.
   ISBN: 1-879384-54-X (pbk.)
   1. Body weight--Regulation. 2. Weight loss. 3. Reducing exercises. 4. Body image. I. Title.
   RA781.6 .H37   2003111154
   613.712--dc22   0312

Manufactured in the USA

2 4 6 8 9 7 5 3 1

First edition

A Note to the Reader

With *Survival of the Thinnest* David Hariton has made a most valuable contribution to our knowledge of the crucially important medical problem of weight control. We were physical animals long before we became thinking ones, and it seems clear that exercise must be of prime importance in one's physiology or how could *Homo sapiens* have survived.

Mr. Hariton maintains that exercise is the key to being thin and that this is genetically determined. He obviously has done his homework and he is an excellent writer, so reading his book was both an instructional and pleasurable experience. I recommend it highly."

— John E. Sarno, M.D.,
author of the best-selling book *Healing Back Pain,* and
Professor of Rehabilitation Medicine at the
New York University School of Medicine

Contents

Introduction

Stop the Endless Dieting Cycle

I WROTE THIS BOOK BECAUSE so many of my friends were having the same frustrating experience that I had until I figured out how to stay thin. At twenty, most of these friends were thin too. Their faces were narrow, angular, and attractive. So were their bodies. You could see their ribs and the shape of their muscles. They had flat stomachs and narrow waists. But over the next twenty years, they gained about a pound of extra weight each year. A layer of fat settled over their faces, destroying the sharpness and angularity of their looks. A thicker layer of fat covered up their muscles, transforming their bodies from objects of beauty to objects of necessity. Bulges appeared and grew on their abdomens, rear ends, and thighs. "Love handles" encircled their waists.

These friends were not lazy, and they were not gluttonous. They struggled with their weight, and they kept going on diets. They avoided snacks, skipped meals, and shunned desserts. They used low-calorie sweetener and low-calorie salad dressing, and had their gravy or sauce "on the side." They pulled the skin off their chicken and cut most of the fat away from their meat. More recently, some of them started removing the bread from their sandwiches and shunning the side dishes on their plates.

Yet all their efforts had surprisingly little effect on their bodies. On one hand, any weight they managed to lose on account of their occasionally radical eating behavior (such as *no* carbohydrates, or *no* fat, or no more than 1,000 calories per day, or even no food at all) came back as soon as they started eating normally again. On the other hand, when they let themselves go and ate whatever they wanted, they didn't become obese. They immediately gained back the few pounds they had lost on their most recent diet, but then their weight stabilized. In fact, it was surprisingly easy for them to maintain a weight that society considered normal for people their age. That weight just happened to be higher than the weight at which they looked their best, and it was a weight at which they were obviously carrying excess fat. What was so frustrating to these people was that they *knew* they could be thin, because they *had* been thin once. What was even more frustrating was that their weight kept creeping up over the years. They would stare in disbelief as the scale reported for the first time that their weight was in the Xs—or as they were forced, for the first time, to buy pants with a size X waist—and they would say to themselves, "This can't be inevitable, since it hasn't even happened before." So they went on dieting.

These people were also not vain. They were leading busy and productive lives, and they had many things that were more important to them than their looks. But the extra fat they were carrying on their bodies hurt their pride, and it therefore made them unhappy. These were people who were admirably in control of everything else in their lives. Why couldn't they control their weight? They didn't have messy homes. They were not sloppy in their careers. They were not careless in their dealings with the people who relied on them. Why were they living in fatty bodies? Life is psychological, and ego plays a central role in it. These people wanted to play the cards they had been dealt as well as they could. One of those cards was their bodies. So they went on dieting.

If you are like these friends of mine, then I have written this book for you, and everything I am about to tell you about how to stay thin will be consistent with your own knowledge and your own experience. It will also be consistent with the results of most research studies and with the advice of most medical experts. The only people it will contradict are the people who advocate various diets to lose the ten to fifty pounds you have gained since you were in college. These people all disagree with each other, and they give contradictory advice. One says to eat pasta and avoid fat. The other says to eat fat and avoid pasta. One says to eat many small, balanced meals. The other says to gorge yourself and then fast. The only thing that all this diet advice has in common is that none of it works—not in the long run.

This book tells you how to stay thin in the long run. It explains why exercise will keep you thin and dieting won't. The explanation is a matter of common sense, given the evolutionary forces that must have shaped our genetic inheritance. But it is an explanation that you're going to have to read to fully grasp. You may not be surprised to discover that people who exercise are thinner than people who don't, but it is important to understand *why* they are thinner, or you won't wind up doing what you need to do to *stay* thin. You may likewise not be surprised to learn that people who go on diets gain all the weight back as soon as they stop, but it is important to understand *why* this happens, or you won't stop wasting your time and effort.

And you *are* wasting your time and effort. You can't stay thin in the long run by fighting your body—by depriving it of food, or of fats, or of car-bohydrates, or by trying to burn off the fat that it is trying so hard to store. It will only rebuild its fat stores as soon as it can, just as it rebuilds other lost body tissues. You've got to focus on the source of your problem: *Why* is your body trying to store more fat, and is there anything you can do to get it to "change its mind"?

This book also explains how exercise can be easier and more fun than dieting, and how it can require far less time and effort than you had imagined. I honestly believe that if you read this book, you will be thin for the rest of your life, and you will be happier and healthier too. I realize there are more important things in life than staying thin. We're lucky to be living in a part of the world where everyone has enough to eat. But taking care of your body is a sensible thing to do, and I see no reason why you should waste your effort on approaches that don't make sense under any analysis. You've spent years rolling a rock up a hill only to watch it slide down again. Give me just an hour or two of your time, and I'm sure I can persuade you to change your approach.

I.

Is Your Body Really Just a Passive Fat Depository?

LET'S START BY TRYING TO ANSWER the question that you've been asking yourself for years. Why is your body storing more and more fat? Why is it doing this *now*, when it didn't do it before?

I am surprised at how rarely people who hope to lose weight speculate about the forces that govern the shapes of their bodies. Why don't people who want to be thinner start by asking themselves why they are not thin right now? They take it for granted that they are no longer thin because they have eaten too much, and that becoming thin again is just a matter of eating less. They view their bodies as passive depositories, like piggy banks. Calories are deposited in the bank when food is consumed. Calories are withdrawn from the bank as energy is expended. The excess of their deposits over their withdrawals equals their fat accounts. To reduce the balance of their fat accounts, they must deposit less, or spend more, or both.

Forgive me, but this doesn't seem like a very thoughtful analysis. Your body is *not* a passive fat depository. It is a life force that actively controls and regulates every aspect of its physical existence. Your body temperature similarly equals the excess of the heat energy you absorb or create over the heat energy that you lose. But if you were running a fever, you wouldn't walk naked through the snow in an effort to lower your body temperature. You would call the doctor to find out *why* your body had raised its temperature. You can't treat an undesirable symptom, like the fact that there is too much fat on your body, by attacking it directly. The symptom will only come back. You must deal with whatever is causing the symptom. Then the symptom will go away by itself.

A great deal of evidence supports the conclusion that your body is actively maintaining its current levels of fat. I could spend the rest of this chapter detailing recent studies of the chemicals, feedback loops, and metabolic adjustments your body employs to accomplish this. But I hope I needn't go into that level of detail to convince you of such an obvious fact. It's a matter of common sense. If your body were just a passive fat depository, if you stayed on a diet you would get thinner and thinner until you died of starvation; and if you never dieted, you would get fatter and fatter until you became grossly obese. Neither of these things happens—not to you, not even to little babies who are allowed to eat as much as they want and never step on a scale. Your body is not relying on you to determine how much fat it should be storing, any more than it is relying on you to determine how much muscle it should be maintaining, or how many blood cells it should be circu-lating, or how many hormones it should be secreting.

Rather, your body has a "lipostat" that is set at a specific level of body fat, just as it has a thermostat that is set at 98.6 degrees. Your body actively *responds* to any sustained variation in caloric intake to maintain the levels of fat that *it* wants to maintain. For example, your body reduces its metabolism in response to a sustained reduction in caloric intake, and it increases its metabolism in response to a sustained increase in caloric intake. Metabolism accounts for 70 percent of an individual's daily caloric expenditure! Your long-term appetite also increases in response to a loss of body fat and decreases in response to an increase in body fat. Your body controls your long-term appetite by varying the levels of appetite-suppressing chemicals, like leptin, that make you feel satiated even though your stomach is empty. Your body also responds to a sustained reduction in caloric intake by producing less thermal energy; discouraging physical activity; increasing psychological interest in appetizing foods; and inducing sensations of hunger in your esophagus and stomach.

It doesn't take much for your body to return its fat levels to where they're set. An energy imbalance of 100 calories per day (the equivalent of an apple, or a light beer) is enough to change your weight by ten pounds over the course of a year. In fact, you are completely dependent on your body's lipostat to maintain your levels of fat in the long run. How could you possibly guess on your own the amount of caloric intake required to regulate your levels of fat so precisely?

How effective can it be, then, to try to force your body to maintain lower levels of fat than it wants to maintain by continually depriving it of food? That's like trying to cool your house by opening the windows while keeping the thermostat at 80 degrees. The heater will respond by generating more heat, and your house will get hot as soon as you close the windows again. The mere fact that you have some short-term control over the level of your fat deposits doesn't mean your body isn't maintaining them in the long run.

You *are* capable of lowering your body temperature in the short run. But if you do, your body will use both physical and psychological means to fight you. It will increase your metabolism, it will generate thermal energy, it will make you shiver, it will make you feel cold, it will make you fantasize about hot fires and warm baths. In the end, you will lose the fight, no matter how determined you are. Why should your experience be any different if you try to maintain lower levels of fat than your body wants you to maintain? Won't it lower your metabolism? Won't it make you feel sensations of hunger, in both your esophagus and your stomach? Won't it make you fantasize about food? I'll bet this has been your experience. I'll bet you gained back most of the weight you lost on your most recent diet, and far sooner than you had hoped. Conversely, the few times in your life when your weight really shot up, I'll bet you had relatively little trouble losing a couple of pounds.

Moreover, when you go on a diet, your body doesn't just consume its stored fat. It also consumes some of its muscle. In effect, it concludes that you need to hold onto your fat, since fat is your most efficient emergency food store, but that you can do without some of the muscle you apparently aren't using. In terms of daily metabolism, muscle is ten times more costly to maintain than fat. No wonder your starving body keeps the fat and gets rid of the muscle. If you were forced to live for ninety days without food, you might survive if your body consumed its muscle first and its fat last, rather than the other way round. But once it consumes its high-metabolism muscle, your body needs less energy to maintain itself, and it becomes that much harder for you to stay thin.

In fact, if you remain sedentary but keep going on diets, you will actually get fatter. Studies show that people who diet store more fat in the long run than people who don't. This is not counterintuitive; it makes perfect sense. According to the body's logic, if you diet you are in greater danger of starvation and need to store more fat as insurance. Studies similarly show that people who dehydrate themselves retain more water, and people who drink water all the time retain less. The body assumes—very logically—that people who often become dehydrated are living in places where water is frequently unavailable, and they are therefore in greater danger of dying of thirst. How depressing for people who try to stay thin by going on diets!

"But if all this is true," you ask, "why was I thin in college? Why was I thinner even five years ago? Don't these facts indicate that my body has no preference regarding how much fat I maintain, at least over a certain range?" No, they don't. What they indicate is that your body's preferences have changed over time. What they indicate is that as you have gotten older and more sedentary, your body has been trying to store more fat. In the next chapter, we try to figure out why. But for now, let's concentrate on why this is the only answer that makes any sense.

Both animals and plants change their physical forms over time to better suit their changing circumstances. Some do so permanently (the caterpillar that turns into a butterfly), some do so seasonally (the bear that stores fat in the fall to prepare for hibernation), and some do so instantaneously (the chameleon that changes color to match its background). But none of these changes is attributable to random forces. Similarly, most of the changes in your own physical form have occurred by design, rather than by default. If you work out or take a job that forces you to lift heavy materials, for example, your muscles increase in size. When you stop, their size decreases again. Your body changes to suit your changing life circumstances.

You grew by several feet when you were a child, but not because that was as fast as you could possibly grow. Some animals grow to sizes that are many times larger in less than a year. The increases in your height and weight were carefully regulated. When you went through puberty, your body changed again. These changes were likewise carefully regulated. If at the same time you lost some of the fat you maintained when you were a child, was that a completely random event? Were you so busy being active, the way kids are, that you forgot to eat enough to maintain your fat deposits? At twenty you were thin, and your weight didn't vary. What happened next? Did your body get lazy? Did it continue to precisely regulate everything about your physical form, from the size and shape of your muscles to the levels of sugar and hormones in your blood, but when it came to your fat deposits, it suddenly threw up its hands and said "Whatever"?

That doesn't make any sense. Your body doesn't let your temperature drift between 93 and 103 degrees. It doesn't allow your muscle tissue to randomly increase or decrease. Your fat is body tissue. Why would your body deal with it differently? To the contrary (as we will soon discuss), for most of the period during which the human race's genes were evolving, the level of our fat deposits was a matter of life or death. It was essential for the body to maintain them at precise and appropriate levels. The logical conclusion is that your body has been trying to store different amounts of fat at different times in your life to suit different life circumstances.

It follows that the reason you are not thin today is *not* because you have been eating too much. It is because you have been eating the right amount. You are not "out of shape" in any objective sense. You are in the shape that your body is actively trying to keep you in. "But how can that be?" I can hear you say. "These love handles? These flabby thighs? This ample rear end? This beer belly? I don't want these things. My companion doesn't want them. Surely my body feels the same way." But your body doesn't have feelings. Your body follows a genetic script. And based on that script, your body is maintaining the size of your love handles just as it maintains the size of your biceps. In following its genetic script, your body does not distinguish among tissues. It does not love your muscles and hate your fat. It maintains the body that biological forces dictate you should have.

Of course you know, from basic biology, that you have a complex genetic inheritance that exists in every cell of your body and that determines almost everything about your body, including the size of your fat deposits. But people tend to have a very static conception of their genetic inheritance. "I got all the fat genes, and my sister got all the thin genes," people are wont to say fatalistically. But it would be far more accurate to conceive of your genetic inheritance as a series of formulas that direct your body to maintain different forms to suit various life circumstances. Consider your genetic inheritance for muscle formation. Do you have "big-muscle genes" or "small-muscle genes"? The answer, of course, is neither. You have a genetic formula that directs your body to increase the size of its muscles when you are lifting a lot of weight and decrease them when you are not. Every mammal on the earth has a genetic inheritance that causes it to adapt its form to suit its changing life circumstances. Have human beings alone inherited forms that are immutable? Have human beings survived and prospered through eons of evolution with bodies that refuse to adapt to their changing life circumstances?

The form your body is trying to maintain is therefore not determined by your genes alone. It is determined by the *interaction* between your genes and your life circumstances. Note that I am not saying you can *fight* your genes by changing your life circumstances. Rather, I'm saying that you *can't* fight your genes, but your genes are not "fat genes" or "thin genes." Your genetic inheritance is directing your body to store fat under some life circumstances and to stay thin under other ones.

Now, one thing we know is that you can't change your genetic inheritance. Although Lamarck once hypothesized that the genes of a giraffe change over time as the giraffe stretches its neck up into the trees to eat leaves, this hypothesis was proven wrong by

Charles Darwin. A giraffe and its offspring will still have the same genes, no matter how much they stretch their necks. But you *can* change your life circumstances. Giraffes do have genes that direct their bodies to maintain longer necks if they stretch them often and shorter necks if they don't. Many of the people I know are like Lamarck. They are convinced that if they keep on dieting, their bodies will give up one day and just keep them thin. But your body doesn't give up, because your genes never change. If you want to stay thin, you're going to have to change your life circumstances and keep them changed.

So what are the life circumstances under which your genetic inheritance will keep you thin? To this we now turn.

2.

Storing Fat Was a Bad Evolutionary Strategy— Except in One Case

I'M ABOUT TO EXPLAIN WHY a person who wants to *stay* thin must stop dieting and start becoming more active. What I'm going to tell you is common sense, yet if you are like most people, you've never even heard it before. And until you hear it—and I mean really hear it—you are never going to do what is necessary to stay thin in the long run. Don't skim this chapter! Read every word, and read it slowly, for while it is important to learn *what* you must do to stay thin, it is more important to understand *why*.

Most of us are carrying a gene that directs our bodies to stay thin while we are active but store fat as soon as we become sedentary. We carry this "active, thin/sedentary, fat" gene because while our species was evolving, storing a lot of fat was a poor evolutionary strategy. Our ancestors had to be exceptionally active—more active than most other large mammals—to successfully pass their genes on to subsequent generations. Storing a lot of fat would have gotten in the way.

But there was one circumstance in which storing more fat did make evolutionary sense. When individuals could not be active—on account of injury, sickness or age—then storing a lot of fat had more benefits than costs. Storing fat didn't prevent such individuals from performing active tasks, since they weren't performing them anyway. But they were presumably incapable of reaching the places where they could forage for food (often at least an hour's walk away), and they were therefore at maximum risk of starvation.

Many people mistakenly assume that our prehistoric ancestors carried an "eat all you can and get as fat as you can, regardless of the circumstances" gene. They assume that the only reason our ancestors didn't get fat is that they never found enough food to eat. If this were true, we would all be fat as houses today. But to help you see how preposterous that is, I'd like to take some time to describe the circumstances under which our genes evolved.

Human beings evolved from apes over the course of several million years, and throughout that period, they were hunter-gatherers. The harsh circumstances that selected most of our genes, including the "active, thin/sedentary, fat" gene, did not abate until 10,000 years ago, with the development of agriculture. The last 10,000 years has not been a long enough or harsh enough period for substantial further evolution to occur (except with respect to immunities from certain rampant diseases). Our bodies today are still governed by our hunter-gatherer genes.

These genes evolved to exploit a migratory existence. The "walking apes" that ultimately evolved into human beings came down out of the trees and forests of Africa to colonize vast grasslands that opened up in response to climatic changes. They relied for their survival on several new capabilities that distinguished them from other apes. One was their ability to dig for tubers, roots, and other food buried beneath the ground; and to reach and gather harder-to-access food above the ground, like nuts, insects, honey, berries, and hard-skinned fruit. Another was their ability to hunt animals on the open savannah, cut their carcasses apart, drag the meat back to temporary camps, and distribute it to their offspring. These abilities allowed the walking apes to occupy habitats that lacked immediately apparent food sources. Other apes were restricted to habitats with low-hanging fruit that immature animals could reach and survive on without assistance from their elders.

Not surprisingly, these new apes evolved a number of features that helped them exploit their new ecology. They initially included an opposable thumb (to grasp tools for digging, hunting, cutting, and carrying food); an upright stance (to free their hands to use these tools, and to free their eyes to spot latent or distant food sources); an efficient bipedal gait emphasizing long-range endurance (to accommodate travel to and from distant food sources); hairlessness (to dissipate heat while traveling to and from distant food sources across the open savannah); prolific sweat glands (a cooling system used in conjunction with hairlessness); a smaller gut (which accommodated greater physical activity and flexibility, but which also required higher-quality food); and a uniquely long postmenopausal lifespan (to help children and grandchildren who were incapable of foraging on their own to reach distant food sources and successfully exploit them). Later, the resulting hominids developed increasingly large and more complex brains, partly to enable them to make and use tools, but equally important, to allow them to figure out and remember where hidden, distant, or migratory food resources were likely to be found, and, through the development of language, to enable them to plan and coordinate the exploitation of those resources.

What is important for our purposes is that all these innovations were designed to exploit an ecology that involved continual travel. Modern African hunter-gatherers change camps to exploit new food resources (and leave resources that have been exhausted) on a monthly basis, and the distance between camps can range up to fifty miles. At any particular camp, clan members of both sexes walk up to two hours in each direction, often pregnant or carrying young children, to reach and exploit the surrounding food resources. They also hunt and scavenge animals, both big and small, and they run to catch up with and capture their prey.

Allow me, then, to make a broad generalization about life during the period in which our genes were evolving. In terms of natural selection, it was *not* a good time to be fat. Survival of the fittest means the survival not of one's self (which always perishes), but the survival of one's children, and of one's children's children.

It didn't matter how abundant the tubers were in a particular month, nor how many animals were caught. All foods were perishable, and it was only a matter of time before the group was likely to travel a great distance to a new food source. Anyone who couldn't make the journey had to be left behind to die, and when an adult died, his or her children and grandchildren probably died as well, since they were not capable of foraging on their own. Moreover, people who were too fat to lead their children or grandchildren to food sources an hour or two from camp were not helping ensure the survival of their genes in subsequent generations. Food sources that were closer to camp were the first to be exhausted, and children who could not reach more distant foraging grounds were the first to die—there was not enough excess food available to support them. The people who arrived first with their children at the site of dwindling food resources were the ones who "survived" in terms of natural selection.

Likewise, anyone who was—
- too fat to pick up a small child and run from a big cat or other predator;
- too fat to dissipate heat while digging for food under the hot African sun;
- too fat to run after potential prey and pursue it for an extended period;
- too fat to reach and scavenge a carcass before it was consumed;
- too fat to run from or after human enemies;
- too fat to join and keep up with a hunting party;
- too fat to get out of the way of large wounded prey;
- too fat to drag a carcass back to hungry children;
- too fat to endure long marches across open fields;
- and too fat to attract the opposite sex

—would not have been likely to leave a lot of genes in subsequent generations.

It is true that fat had an important advantage: it allowed the person who carried it to survive longer without food. Food sources were variable, and people were sometimes incapacitated. There was therefore an optimum amount of fat that our genes directed even active people to carry on their bodies to minimize their risk of starvation. For men, this appears to be (in addition to "vital" fat, like the fat on your heart) about 10 percent of their body weight, and for women, about 20 percent of their body weight. The additional fat stored on women may have served as a special reserve for pregnancy and lactation. Women also needed more fat because they had less muscle to consume and survive on when food was unavailable. Some anthropologists speculate that given its typical placement on the rear end and thighs, this extra fat also helped women balance the weight of the babies they carried inside or outside their bodies so they could maintain the all-important efficiency and long-range endurance of their bipedal gait.

In any case, these were optimum levels of fat because (along with consumable muscle tissue) they generally allowed people to survive without any food at all for sixty to ninety days (stored fat is a very efficient source of energy).

Up to these levels, the storage of body fat increased an individual's fitness in evolutionary terms. But beyond these levels, it decreased the individual's fitness, because it got in the way of efforts to perform vital tasks for children and to dissipate heat. Bear in mind that the great famines that have been the scourge of recent human existence did not occur prior to the advent of agriculture. Once agriculture was introduced, relatively small amounts of land could support millions of people, and when crops failed, those millions of people had no other means of subsistence. But until then, those same lands could support only thousands of people. If the March berry bushes were sparse one year, people could look for berries elsewhere, or go hunting instead. Sickness and injury (such as a broken leg) were the most likely sources of temporary privation. But the ability to lead children to food and to fight off or escape predators (especially large cats) was probably more important, in evolutionary terms, than the ability to survive for months on end without food.

The only time, then, when it made evolutionary sense to store a lot of fat was when an individual had been incapacitated by injury, sickness, or age. Such an individual was not worthless in evolutionary terms. An incapacitated individual could still care for young children and grandchildren; make tools, clothing, and shelters; store or prepare food; and protect the camp from predators. In the struggle with the forces of natural selection, any act that increased the likelihood of survival of one's children and grandchildren furthered the propagation of one's own genetic makeup, and the survival of even an older person was therefore genetically important. But an incapacitated individual could not reach foraging grounds and had to rely on excess food brought back by others. The availability of such food was erratic, to say the least. And since the individual's ability to run or walk long distances was in such circumstances irrelevant, a "fit" gene would have directed the individual's body to store more fat, rather than allow excess food (which could not be stored in a refrigerator or freezer) to go to waste.

For most of the millions of years during which our genes evolved, our ancestors lived in Africa. They colonized the rest of the world only over the course of the last 100,000 years. (Close cousins of ours appeared outside Africa as much as a million years ago, but they all died out and were replaced by the *Homo sapiens* that colonized the world more recently.) This may not, in any case, have been a long enough period to evolve substantially different fat-maintenance genes, but the evolutionary forces that our ancestors encountered in their new environments still selected *for* the "active, thin/sedentary, fat" gene. Survival on the plains of Europe revolved around the hunting of large migratory animals, and it therefore demanded speed, endurance, and the ability to dissipate heat.

Moreover, as they began to encounter a winter period during which the earth was covered with snow and ice, human beings had to withdraw seasonally to warmer climates, and this forced them to walk long distances at least twice a year, carrying children and tools. Alternatively, some of them may have adopted a winter survival strategy under which young people traveled great distances to hunt for game, while nursing women, children, and older people remained behind in camp, performing more sedentary tasks. Because the ground was covered with ice, children could not forage for food directly, and the group was wholly dependent on whatever food the hunting party managed to bring back. It would have been all the more important for the members of such a temporarily sedentary group to store fat while they had the opportunity to do so (when the hunters had a streak of good luck). But these members would have wanted to shed any residual fat in the spring, when food was available and general activity began again, and the young hunters certainly wouldn't have wanted to store a lot of fat. What more adaptive gene could there be for such a group than the "active, thin/sedentary, fat" gene?

It is true that the weather was colder, but animals requiring insulation develop body hair or fur, not fat. Storing fat is a relatively costly and ineffective means of retaining heat. The purpose of fat is to provide an emergency energy store. Extremely cold weather selects for stockier bodies and limbs that limit exposure to the cold and resist frostbite, not for increased body fat. Eskimos living traditional lives are not fat, and their ability to retain heat correlates with their compact body proportions, not with increased fat deposits. In any case, human beings had warm animal skins, shelters, and fire to help them retain heat. It was more important for them to be able to *dissipate* heat when they had to.

In other words, the assumption that our genes tell us to consume all the food we can fit into our stomachs, regardless of the circumstances, is not logical in light of our evolutionary history. Our genetic inheritance was shaped by harsh environmental forces. Our biological ancestors were constantly making tradeoffs among competing evolutionary objectives: to procreate with a fit mate, to help children and grandchildren find food, and to avoid predators (including other humans). The forms of their bodies were not a matter of personal preference; they were a matter of life and death, of success or failure in the struggle to pass genes on to subsequent generations. Surely they were not randomly determined by how much food our ancestors happened to come across and how much they enjoyed eating.

And since our genes have not changed very much since then, I doubt that people today are storing more fat than they want to store because they have been overwhelmed by the pleasure of eating. The biological reality is precisely the opposite: we experience eating as pleasurable *because* it is necessary to maintain our physical forms. Most individuals find eating irresistible until they reach the levels of fat their bodies want them to maintain, and then their weight stabilizes. But that doesn't mean they are maintaining the levels of fat they desire. Consider the biological maxim, "Form follows function." If you are primarily sedentary, your genetic inheritance causes your body to store more fat than you want it to store. Your genetic inheritance doesn't know that the Stone Age is over.

Many people also assume that the people in third-world countries stay thin because they do not have the *opportunity* to get fat, but common sense belies this assumption as well. Except in times of famine, plenty of starchy food is available in most third-world countries. If people in such countries were staying thin merely because they couldn't find enough food, they would by definition be on the edge of starvation. The richest people would be fat, the poorer people would be thin but barely surviving, and the poorest people would be dying of starvation. World populations become fatter not as their capacity to produce food increases, but rather as they become more *sedentary*. They get fatter to the extent that they replace walking and bicycling with motor-biking and driving, start buying washing machines and televisions, and replace manual labor with office jobs.

Likewise, many people assume that our children are gaining weight because they are eating too many carbohydrates. (The percentage of children with excess fat reserves has risen in some first-world countries from 7 to 25 percent of the population.) But do we really think our children's bodies are suddenly malfunctioning? Have our remarkable bodies, which fight diseases using methods too complex for even our greatest scientists to understand, really been defeated by encounters with corn syrup and starch? Our children are, in fact, eating more protein and less starch than those of prior generations. What they are doing that's new is spending most of their free time watching television and playing Nintendo games, rather than playing sports and running around outdoors. Every available study relates the recent increase in childhood obesity to the recent increase in sedentary behavior among children. The prehistoric genes of these children are telling their bodies to store fat because they are apparently not in a position to go out and forage for food. As far as their bodies can tell, these children are eating food that other people have foraged for them.

In fact, most human beings, regardless of their origin, carry the "active, thin/sedentary, fat" gene. Studies involving individuals, twins, identical twins, groups, and world populations all show that active people become and remain thinner than sedentary people. Evidence from studies involving pets and animals in captivity suggests that the "active, thin/sedentary, fat" gene is (for similar reasons) prevalent in the mammalian population at large.

Are there any *other* genetic formulas that help us survive pre-historic living conditions by increasing or decreasing our levels of body fat? Suppose that someone eats relatively little food for several weeks and then starts eating full meals again. Wouldn't an evolu-tionarily successful gene direct the body to store more fat under such circumstances, to better suit the unpredictable nature of that individual's food sources? After all, prehistoric people didn't read diet books. If they were not eating enough to maintain the levels of fat that their bodies wanted them to maintain, it was because food was unavailable. Conversely, if someone was eating enough, it was because that individual was in close proximity to food, probably out hunting and gathering, rather than waiting in camp for someone else to bring food back. Such a person would be less likely to face privation for an extended period, so it would be less important for that person to store fat as a safety measure.

Imagine, if you will, two genetic formulas competing with each other over the course of eons to determine which one survives in subsequent generations. The first one effectively says, "If you have starved until you have lost most of your fat stores, then rebuild those fat stores as soon as you can and add some more on for good measure." The second one effectively says, "If you have starved until you have lost most of your fat stores, keep them off—you look marvelous!" Which formula would you expect to have successfully replicated itself in subsequent generations? Which formula would you expect to find governing human body forms today?

Suppose that a person's muscles have atrophied from lack of use. That person would have more need for fat, because muscle and fat both serve as emergency food reserves. That person would also have more room for fat. Conversely, if an active person *must* have more muscle to perform vital daily activities, then that person doesn't need as much fat and doesn't have as much room for fat. Wouldn't an evolutionarily successful genetic formula therefore be, "If the body has more muscle, store less fat"? Consider the alternative genetic formula, "Store fat on an active body without regard to how much muscle the body is already carrying." Which of these two formulas would you expect to have replicated itself in successive generations and to be governing human body forms today?

Alas, we are probably also carrying a gene that directs a sedentary body to store more fat as it ages. During the period in which human genes were evolving, teenagers were engaged in the all-important task of finding a mate for procreation. The more fit (in evolutionary terms) were the mates they attracted, the more fit were the children they produced, the better those children would be provided for, and the more likely they would be to survive and produce fit children of their own. It was therefore probably more important, in evolutionary terms, for even a lame teenager to look good than to store fat.

But it was probably far more important for a mother in her thirties to survive than to look good. If she died, her children and grandchildren were likely to die with her. Her survival strategy was not to attract a fit mate to produce more children (as her impending menopause would soon emphasize) but rather to look after the children she had already had. And if she was sedentary, her best survival strategy was to store more fat. Form follows function.

Well, what does all this say about the interaction between our genetic inheritance and our life circumstances? The message is obvious. A person who wants to *stay* thin must stop dieting and start becoming more active. What little remains of Paleolithic art (stone figurines and so forth) suggests that the only people who were fat during the Stone Age were revered tribal chiefs and queens. These people presumably did not forage for themselves but rather had food brought back to them by others. Today we are all tribal chiefs and queens, and we are going to have to turn back into commoners if we want to stay thin.

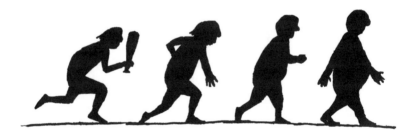

"But I can't be active all day," I can hear you saying. "I have a sedentary job. I have kids to take care of. That's how *I* survive." The good news is that you don't *have* to be active all day. You just have to convince your body that there is something you must do on a daily basis that requires speed and endurance, and it therefore can't *afford* to store a lot of fat. The fact that your body doesn't "understand" modern society is a blessing as well as a curse. It may be true that your body doesn't understand, when you go on a diet, that you are not in danger of starvation, but it also doesn't understand, when you maintain an elevated heart rate, that you really don't have to. It will effectively assume that you are running (there were no exercise machines in the Stone Age), for reasons that are important in evolutionary terms (for instance, this is how you obtain food for your children), and it will change its shape accordingly. Form follows function.

The next chapter tells you how to turn on your "active/thin" gene with the minimum amount of time and effort. It tells you how you can persuade your body that it can't afford to store fat, without turning your life upside down. Of course you won't really be misleading your body, because it *doesn't* need to store a lot of fat. The point is that your genetic inheritance is not telling your body to store fat regardless of the circumstances. It is telling your body to store fat if it can without interfering with other, more important evolutionary objectives. Your business is to persuade your body that it *can't*.

Before we leave prehistoric times, I'd like to offer you one last thought. Could convincing your body that you still need to be active have beneficial effects apart from keeping you thin? Could it also serve to slow the process of mental and physical deterioration? Some geneticists have speculated that there is a reason, apart from wear and tear, why degeneration and disease occur primarily in older people: younger people have not yet raised their children to the point where they can survive on their own. A successful genetic formula would obviously have kept degeneration at bay until this all-important survival task had been completed. But this job would not necessarily have been completed merely because an individual had gotten older. If an older person was out hunting, gathering, and leading children and grandchildren to food, those activities would have been vital to the survival of that person's genetic inheritance. Such a situation would likely have coincided with a late birth or with the early death of a parent, in which case the relevant children might have starved without the older person's performance. But if older people were completely sedentary (not even making tools and shelters), then as an evolutionary matter they were, to put it bluntly, expendable. Such people were really just taking up space, and eating up food, that would have been better reserved for their offspring, so that their genetic inheritance could be passed on. An evolutionarily successful gene might therefore have directed their bodies not to struggle so hard against degenerative forces.

Sound far-fetched? Perhaps so. And being thin and fit is reward enough for exercising. But studies have shown that increased physical activity reduces the frequency and severity of most chronic diseases that are associated with aging, including heart and artery disease, strokes, some forms of cancer, osteoporosis, and diabetes. And I have friends who claim that the process of deterioration in their elderly parents seemed to accelerate when they stopped being mentally and physically active or lost their sense of purpose.

3.

How to Make Your Body Think You Run for a Living

IF YOU CONSISTENTLY PERFORM thirty minutes per day of aerobic exercise, you will—over the course of several months—become as thin and toned as you were when you were in your twenties, without dieting or otherwise obsessing over food. And you will stay that way for as long as you continue exercising. You will also be happier, healthier, and more energetic. You don't believe me? Try it for just a few months.

When you perform aerobic exercise, your body assumes you are running. Prehistoric people rarely ran for the fun of it. Running is very costly as a biological matter. It causes the body to generate excess heat that it must dissipate by pumping blood to the surface of the skin. It also pounds the delicate joints and muscles of the legs, and a barefoot runner can step on sharp rocks, branches, or other objects and become injured or infected. Human beings are among the least efficient runners in the animal kingdom. A prehistoric human who ran for an extended period was doing so for only one reason: to catch food and bring it home to hungry children. Despite the sloth and inefficiency of their running gait, prehistoric humans were superb *endurance* hunters. Their remarkable ability to dissipate heat allowed them to play the tortoise to their prey's hare. Their prey had to stop running after relatively short sprints, because their bodies became overheated. But the human hunters kept on coming, and eventually they caught up.

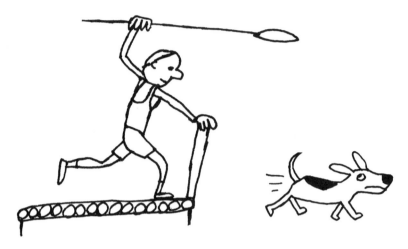

The object of your exercise is to persuade your body that you are one of those hunters. It is to persuade your body that you *must* maintain an elevated heart rate to feed your hungry family. Then your body will do whatever it can to help you succeed. And the first thing it can do to help you succeed is to get rid of your excess fat stores. Biologically, it is relatively efficient for a sedentary person to carry excess fat around. The body expends only a tenth as much energy to maintain fat as it expends to maintain an equivalent amount of muscle mass. But it is very hard for a person to run long distances while carrying excess fat. Not only does the excess fat force the body to drag more weight along, but it also makes it much harder for the body to dissipate heat. There are some pretty chubby professional baseball players around, but how many fat basketball or tennis players have you seen running up and down the court?

Now I can already hear you saying, "I *have* tried aerobic exercise, and it didn't work for me." But I'm willing to bet that you didn't do it long enough, consistently enough, and energetically enough to give your body the message that it can't afford to store fat. Occasional exercise and moderate exercise will not suffice to keep you thin. Such exercise may use up a little bit of your fat stores, but your body will quickly replenish them. A single soft drink will replace the calories it has burned. If you want to persuade your body that it shouldn't be storing fat, you must exercise every day, and you must not stop doing it. I don't care if you run marathons, climb mountains, or go on bicycle hikes. If you are not making aerobic exercise a part of your *daily* life, then you are not sending your body the "I can't afford to store fat" message.

Studies generally bear this out. People who exercise only a few times per week, or who exercise at low to moderate intensity levels, do not maintain low levels of body fat. Some studies have been designed to support the argument that a little bit of exercise is better than nothing. The people conducting these studies reason as follows: "We can't persuade people to perform aerobic exercise every day. Let's at least try to persuade them to take a walk once in a while and get up to change the TV channel." I don't doubt that occasional or moderate exercise is better than nothing, but it is not enough to keep you from storing fat, and the evidence is clear.

What's more, it is not easier to make occasional exercise a habit. It's harder, because neither you nor your body gets used to it. A habit is precisely that: something you do all the time. When you exercise every day, your body gradually changes in physical and psychological ways that make it easy for you to perform the task that you apparently must perform. Your fat cells learn to release sugar into your bloodstream; your muscles learn to take in more sugar and oxygen and produce more energy; your heart becomes stronger; your body secretes chemicals that suppress any sensations of displeasure; and most important, your mind learns how to make you *want* to perform that which survival apparently requires. But if you don't exercise every day, your body will realize that your exercise isn't necessary, and then it will do whatever it can to get you to stop. It will make you dread the very thought of exercise. After all, running is biologically inefficient, so your body doesn't want you to do it unless you *have* to.

Besides, there are other good reasons to exercise every day. Being in shape is a sensual delight. It allows you play tennis, go hiking, bound up stairs, enjoy long walks, run whenever you want to, and otherwise conduct an active life with ease. Daily exercise improves your health and decreases your risk of heart and circulatory disease. And daily exercise gives you a psychological lift. You don't just feel more energetic. You feel more cheerful, more positive, and more competent. Researchers have found that exercise causes the body to release certain chemicals into the bloodstream as part of its fight-or-flight response, and these chemicals produce a sense of energy, focus, and euphoria. Many psychologists recommend exercise to alleviate depression.

Monitoring Your Heart Rate

When I say the daily exercise you perform must be aerobic exercise, I mean it must consume a lot of oxygen and therefore give your body the message that you are running. Such exercise substantially increases your heart rate because your heart must pump all this oxygen to your muscles. Your heart rate is, in fact, a direct measure of the amount of oxygen you are consuming (except during the first few minutes of your exercise). You therefore want to rely on your heart rate to determine the pace of your exercise. For any given level of exercise, both your oxygen consumption and your heart rate vary from day to day, and even from minute to minute, depending on your sugar levels, digestion, hormone levels, fatigue, stress, mental activity, and body temperature. Your body temperature in turn depends on such external factors as the ambient temperature, humidity, and breeze. You want to keep your heart rate steady and vary your exercise level, not the other way around.

You can purchase an inexpensive wristwatch heart monitor at most sporting goods stores. If you haven't yet had time to buy one, measure your pulse while exercising by following these simple steps: First, gently press your fingers against your heart or your carotid artery (at the top of the side of your neck, just below your jaw, where you would normally feel your glands). Second, slow your pace momentarily to match your pulse (so that your count doesn't get confused)—that is, one stride, or stroke, or rotation per beat of your heart. Third, look at your watch and note how many strides, or strokes, or rotations you perform in the course of fifteen seconds. Fourth, multiply the result by four. The answer you get may not be precise, but it will give you a pretty good sense of where you are.

It is unfortunately not possible for me to tell you what your target heart rate should be. (In fact, I don't even know if you should be exercising—be sure to read the disclaimer at the end of this chapter.) Resting heart rates can vary substantially among individuals. You may therefore have to rely partly on how your body feels when you exercise. Try jogging gently for five or ten minutes. You are seeking an exercise level that feels the same way. You certainly shouldn't be exercising too hard, and I generally don't allow my heart rate to climb above 155 beats per minute. But your exercise must not feel like a walk in the park, either. Even after you are in shape, there should still be some part of your body that, if you listened to it, would seem to be saying, "Do you mind if we stop now? Wouldn't you rather be lounging about?" The physical sensation that carries this message may change over time, but if the only reason part of you would prefer to stop is that you're feeling bored, then you are not exercising hard enough.

Once you are in shape, you can use your in-shape resting heart rate to determine your target heart rate with more precision. (Don't try doing this before you're in shape. Your current resting heart rate may be twenty beats higher than it will be once you get in shape, and you don't want to exercise at a rate that is twenty beats too high!) The approach that works best for me is called the Karvonen method, and it is based on the difference between your resting heart rate and your maximum heart rate. This method advocates exercising in a range that is between 70 and 80 percent of that difference. Your in-shape resting heartbeat is something you'll have to measure. Be sure you are really resting when you do. Sit still in a chair for several minutes first. You may need the help of a physical therapist to measure your maximum heart rate, but a good working assumption is that your maximum heart rate equals 220 minus your age, which is 175 beats per minute for a forty-five-year-old like me.

Allow me to demonstrate the Karvonen method by applying it to myself. My in-shape resting heart rate happens to be 66. I assume that my maximum heart rate is 175. The difference between these two figures is 109 (175 – 66). The range between 70 and 80 percent of this difference is 76 to 87 beats per minute. I must add my resting heartbeat to this range to figure out my target exercise range. This means I should exercise in a range between 142 (76 + 66) and 153 (87 + 66) beats per minute. And that, indeed, is what I do.

Because my maximum heart rate slows down as I get older (I assume that it is 220 minus my age), my exercise range likewise gets lower as I get older. Under the Karvonen method, I would have aimed to exercise in a range between 149 and 161 when I was thirty-five, and I will aim to exercise in a range between 135 and 145 when I am fifty-five. Please also bear in mind that I use an exercise bike. Friends who use certain elliptical machines have lower target heart rates because they are using their arms as well as their legs. Some of my friends have lower heart rates, period. I never allow my heart rate to fall below 140 while exercising, but it is perfectly possible for you to be my age and have a target heart rate of 135.

Naturally, your heart rate will not jump up to 140 (or whatever your target heart rate is) as soon as you start your exercise. It will rise steadily over the course of several minutes and then reach a plateau. Later on, it may start drifting upward again (so-called cardiac drift) as your body builds up heat and your heart pumps more blood to the surface of your skin to cool you down. Exercise vigorously enough at first to reach your plateau within a few minutes, and then vary your pace or level to maintain a steady elevated heart rate for the remainder of your exercise period.

What Sort of Exercise Should I Do?

Your exercise should primarily involve your leg muscles, since they are larger than your arm muscles and consume more oxygen. In a moment we will consider some of the principal alternatives. But choose the exercise that is easiest and most comfortable for you to perform and that you enjoy the most. In other words, choose the exercise that you are most likely to stick to on a permanent basis. You should also have a backup exercise that doesn't involve a machine (so you can perform it when you are away on a trip) and that uses a different group of muscles than your principal exercise does, in case one of your muscles gets sore. Be sure to perform your backup exercise often enough to keep the relevant muscles in shape. Otherwise, you'll be sore whenever you try it.

Exercise Machines

Exercise machines have a lot of advantages. They generally allow you to perform a balanced exercise that uses more of your muscle groups. This minimizes the strain on any particular muscle and helps you avoid soreness, wear and tear, and injury. It also makes your exercise easier and more enjoyable to perform. Beginners who give in to the temptation to stop often do so in response to a complaining muscle. But your muscles are less likely to complain when you are on a good exercise machine. You also may not have to stretch as much, and this will save you some time.

Exercising on a machine can be convenient and flexible, especially if you can afford to purchase one and keep it at home or if there is one in a gym down the hall at work. Many machines allow you to perform other constructive tasks, like reading or work, while exercising. An indoor machine lets you exercise in any kind of weather. And a machine makes it easier to maintain your target heart rate in a controlled and steady fashion by adjusting your exercise level.

Many exercise machines report your heart rate to you on a continuous basis. This saves you the trouble of having to buy and wear independent monitoring equipment. But note that many exercise machines also have charts on them suggesting different heart rates for different age groups. These charts usually have a lower "fat-burning range" and a higher "cardio-training range." You want to be close to the top of the higher "cardio-training range." You do *not* want to be in the lower fat-burning range, because, as we've discussed, you can't fight your body by burning off the fat it is trying so hard to store. The reason you are exercising is to send your body the message that fat is something it cannot afford to store. Likewise, pay no attention to your "calories burned," your "speed," your "watts," your "calories per hour," or any of the other helpful pieces of information that the machine may offer you from time to time. They have nothing to do with your objective. Similarly, do *not* select one of the preplanned courses of exercise that purport to be taking you up hills and down dales. Your objective is not to simulate a trip to the seaside. It is to maintain your pulse at a constant elevated rate.

If you are currently inactive, you will be starting out at a relatively low exercise level, because that will suffice to increase the rate of your out-of-shape heart. Don't feel frustrated or impatient. You are accomplishing everything you need to accomplish. Your heart and muscles will quickly get stronger, and you will therefore be forced to increase your exercise level to maintain your target rate. At some point, though, you will plateau at an exercise level that is appropriate for your new, in-shape body. When this happens, don't feel disappointed that you are no longer making "progress" and start pushing yourself beyond your capabilities. You are not accomplishing any less than you were accomplishing before.

Exercise machines can simulate anything from climbing stairs to cross-country skiing. You should try out different machines at a local gym. But once you know the kind you like, I urge you to buy one for use in your home, even if you can only afford a less expensive model. For the biggest problem with exercise machines is that most people have to go to the gym to use them, and that turns daily exercise into a federal case. You have to travel to the gym, change your clothes, go up and exercise, go back down to the locker room, take a shower, get dressed again, and travel back to your home or place of work. You may even have to wait for someone else to get off your favorite exercise machine. All this takes up a lot of time. No wonder most people don't exercise every day. Most people are very busy. So if you can't afford to buy an exercise machine—and you work, have children, or both—you might want to consider something else.

An excellent group of exercise machines that have become very popular of late are generically called elliptical machines. They generally let you perform a movement that is something in between jogging, bicycling, climbing, and cross-country skiing. This motion allows you to use more muscle groups (including, in some cases, your arm muscles), and this serves both to reduce the strain on any particular muscle group and to produce better overall muscle conditioning. Unfortunately, it is difficult to acquire the best machines for home use, because they are large, have unattractive frames, and tend to be very expensive. I myself still use a stationary exercise bike, partly because I have gotten used to it. Stationary bikes are compact, relatively inexpensive, and even relatively attractive. When I am traveling, I can find one in most hotels or local gyms. They don't make me sweat very much, and I find it easy to read or do my work on them. More important, for some reason I find their cycling motion easy to perform for an extended period. I prefer the kind that resembles a bicycle, but some people prefer the recumbent kind that lets you kick your legs out in front of you as you pedal. The advantage is that it puts less pressure on your groin and rear end, but the disadvantage is that it forces you to hold your legs up while pedaling.

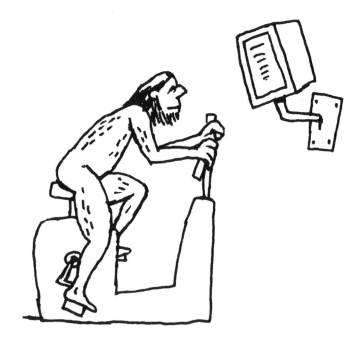

Other people favor jogging on an indoor treadmill, but I'm not sure why. Jogging outdoors can be wonderful, as we are about to discuss, but no matter how gently you jog, you are still pounding your knees, ankles, and joints, and jostling your muscles and tendons. Why do this when you are indoors anyway, and another machine will produce results that are just as good?

Outdoor Jogging

Jogging outdoors allows you to watch the scenery change while you take command of your body and radiate energy. If you are lucky enough to be in the country, it lets you access the beauty of nature. On clear days, the sunlight may stream through the trees. The ocean may roar at your side. The birds may call to one another above your head. Soft breezes may blow to charm you. If it is early morning, as it should be for reasons I explain below, then it will be cool, and you will pretty much have the world to yourself. No cars will pass to annoy or distract you. No people will giggle or shout. The long rays of morning light will wend their way up the trunks of trees and along the roadside, inviting your eye to follow them. But even in the city, outdoor exercise reveals some of the beauty you've been missing in the city's composed and varied landscapes.

Jogging is also something you can do anywhere. You won't have to find your way to a gym, and if you exercise before your morning shower, you won't have to shower and dress twice.

For younger people, jogging has two advantages over the fast walking that I discuss further below. First, it is difficult to jog too slowly, so jogging is a good way for a younger person to be sure to maintain a high enough heart rate. Second, jogging is a more natural motion to perform at aerobic speeds, and many younger people therefore prefer it. But unlike fast walking, jogging pounds your legs into the ground. I therefore recommend that anyone who jogs on a daily basis do so thoughtfully and carefully. Never lose sight of your objective, which is to stay thin. This means you must exercise in a manner that allows you to perform your exercise every day and maintain your target heart rate with the minimum wear, tear, and effort.

Here are my ten jogging do's and don'ts:

1. Maintain a slow and steady pace, measuring your heart rate from time to time to be sure it isn't too fast. I use the word "jog" because that is all it should be—the next step up from a fast walk.

Jogging outdoors is not a competition. If you are jogging with a competitive friend, let the friend run on ahead. Don't return home bragging to yourself that you have just jogged four, or six, or eight miles. How far or how fast you've jogged is irrelevant to your purpose. Your only purpose is to maintain your target heart rate while avoiding injury.

2. Take moderate strides, and keep your feet low to the ground. Don't go leaping through the air and landing with a thud, as if you thought you were Barishnikov. The smaller your strides, the easier it is to control them. Maintain good form, landing on your heel and rotating forward so that you push off from the ball of your foot. Never land on the front of your foot. Try to land as softly as you can, to protect the delicate tendons and carefully formed joints of your feet, calves, knees, and thighs. Set aside your fear that you don't look cool enough. The world is really not watching us, even though we may think it is.

3. Be sure to vary your pace to match your terrain. When you are jogging uphill, slow down to be sure you are not using more energy than you use to run on flat ground. On a steep hill, you should almost be jogging in place, while pushing upward with your calf and rear end muscles, as if you were climbing stairs. Otherwise, you will needlessly stress your heart and tire your leg muscles, making the rest of your jog more difficult and making it more likely that you will be tempted to stop. The only change you should notice while you are jogging uphill is that your calves are doing more work while your thighs are doing less. The jog should not feel harder to perform. Similarly, increase your speed when you are jogging downhill. Don't increase it so much that you lose control, of course, and bear in mind that resisting your own gravity also requires energy. Be sure to check your heart monitor on sustained downward or upward inclines to help you modify your pace. Also, don't hesitate to avoid hills altogether by turning around and jogging back and forth along a level stretch.

4. Don't stop. If you must wait for a traffic light or say hello to a friend, continue to jog in place so that your heart rate doesn't fall. There's nothing wrong with jogging in place—it's a perfectly viable form of aerobic exercise.

5. Jog on a flat, smooth surface, like a road, boardwalk, or well-mown lawn. Don't jog across a field or along the beach. If you insist on beach jogging, at least jog where the water has made the sand hard. But even jogging on hard sand will needlessly add to the burden of your ankles and calves.

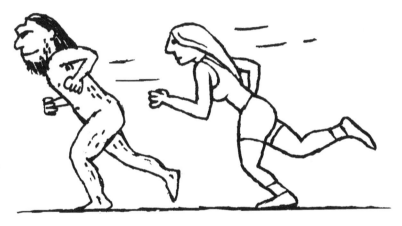

6. Be sure to stretch your leg muscles before and after you jog, especially after.

7. Buy and wear good running shoes. Support is very important, and you're not going to be able to jog for years if you don't take care of your feet.

8. Don't jog every day. Do something else twice each week, to give your jogging muscles a rest. In any case, always switch to your backup exercise if your leg muscles feel tired or sore. Listen to your legs and believe them when they tell you they need a rest. If you start receiving signals of mild pain midway through your jog, switch to fast walking immediately, or stop altogether if necessary. It is true that the mild pain will go away if you keep on jogging, but

you felt the pain for a reason. Your legs were in effect saying, "Yes, we can go on if we must, but this is costing us, and we are going to have to spend some time recovering." Don't assume that this is impossible just because you've been jogging every day without a problem. The effects of jogging are cumulative, and there will be some days when one of your muscles has simply had enough. If you push your muscles beyond their capabilities, your body may convince you to stop exercising altogether. So switch to another exercise before you switch to nothing at all.

9. Don't get "into" running if you want to use jogging as your principal form of exercise. Don't make friends with runners and compete with them. Don't start trying to go further and faster. Above all, *don't* train for and run marathons. All you will accomplish by doing these things is to damage the joints and muscles you are relying on for your daily exercise. It goes without saying that if you run a marathon, you won't even be able to jog every day for a while. If you enjoy running marathons or running as a sport (which is perfectly fine, of course), then pick something else, like an exercise machine, for your daily exercise.

The following is an exchange I sometimes have with running enthusiasts who are not as thin as they would like to be:

Me: If you want to say thin, you have to perform aerobic exercise on a daily basis.

Runner: I tried that. It doesn't work.

Me: Have you really tried it?

Runner: Are you kidding? I run marathons!

Me: Yes, but have you tried daily aerobic exercise?

It invariably turns out that these people train for marathons, but once they get through them, they are so exhausted that they live sedentary lives for several months. Even while they are training, they don't run every day. What did they think was going to happen to them when they stopped running? Did they think their bodies would be so impressed with them for running a marathon that they would forget to store fat when they became incapacitated?

10. Don't try jogging if you are an exercise beginner. With jogging it is impossible to start out slowly, and you are therefore more likely to quit before you have a chance to get in shape. It is also harder on your muscles, and the ache of sore muscles will discourage you. An exercise machine will let you start at a lower level and avoid soreness while you work yourself into shape. After a month or two, you'll be ready to switch over to jogging, if that is what you prefer.

Fast Walking

Fast (or aerobic) walking is one of the best forms of exercise. The first thing to bear in mind about fast walking, though, is that *you mustn't kid yourself*. It's easy to slack off while walking fast, and you must really push yourself to maintain your target heart rate. The rule is the opposite of the one that applies to jogging: you must go as fast as you can (except when you are going uphill). In terms of pace, fast walking should feel like jogging, and to get a better sense of it, you should try jogging slowly and then extending your legs out in front of you to transition into fast walking, without losing significant speed.

The motion of walking is not as natural as jogging when it is performed at aerobic rates, and it will seem awkward at first. Fast walking is *not* the same as mere brisk walking. In brisk walking you mainly use your calf muscles, but in fast walking you also rely on your thigh, rear end and back muscles to propel your body powerfully forward. If you're not used to fast walking, your muscles will complain at first, and yes, they may be sore for several days afterward. In other words, fast walking is an aerobic exercise that uses all the muscles of your lower body; brisk walking is not. You cannot maintain your target heart rate with brisk walking, and if you don't, you will not be accomplishing the principal purpose of your exercise, which is to keep you thin.

Of course, outdoor fast walking offers all the pleasures that outdoor jogging does. And since it doesn't pound your legs, I recommend it over jogging for older people and people with sensitvie muscles or joints. If you wish, you can alternate between fast walking and slow jogging, so that you give different muscles a workout and minimize your risk of soreness. But be sure to follow all the applicable do's and don'ts set out above for jogging. For example, if you are walking fast in the city and have to stop for oncoming traffic, be sure to switch from walking to jogging in place. You should never allow yourself to simply stand still.

Proper form is also important. Don't try to take giant strides. It's the number of strides you take per minute that matters, not their size. Try to glide along in a continuous motion, as if you were bicycling, rather than hiking. Keep your body almost erect and your head up and looking ahead. Don't lean out in front of your stride or look down at the ground. Relax any muscles that aren't performing. Don't make a fist, grit your teeth, or tense your neck or shoulder muscles.

Try to make your feet follow a straight line. Push off of the middle of the toes of your back foot with your back leg slightly bent, while extending your front leg fully out in front of you. Land on the heel of your front foot, with your toes pointed straight ahead, and simultaneously pull your forward heel down toward you (that is, into the ground), effectively using it as a fulcrum to propel yourself forward, so that the shin of your forward leg also does some of the work. Allow each hip to move down and then up (not side to side) as each leg moves forward and then back.

Keep your elbows bent at a 90-degree angle, and allow your arms to swing forward and back. You may allow them to swing in at an angle toward (but not across) the middle of your chest. But don't let your elbows drift up and out to your side, as if you were flapping your wings; and don't swing your arms higher than 90 degrees, as if you were a drum major.

Jogging Indoors, Aerobics, and Other Backup Exercises

Outdoor exercise may be unpleasant if it is cold outside or raining. But what are your alternatives? This can be a pressing question when you are away on vacation or a business trip and no gym is available.

Once you have gotten used to jogging, you can actually jog anywhere. You can jog in a circle around a room, you can jog back and forth down a hallway, or you can even just jog in place. (If you're in a high-rise, let's hope your floors have carpeting, for the sake of your downstairs neighbor.) To the extent that you are not propelling yourself forward, however, you will be relying solely on your calf muscles (and not on your thigh muscles) to perform your exercise. Your calf muscles will likely become sore if you jog in place for thirty minutes when you aren't used to it.

Another alternative is to perform a series of repetitive exercises for no more than a few minutes each, so that none of your muscles gets sore. These exercises can include stepping back and forth in different directions, hopping, skipping, kicking, or jumping, all while throwing your arms up into the air in different directions. They can also involve stepping onto, and off of, a platform. You can take a class at most gyms to learn some of these aerobic exercises or buy a book describing them. It doesn't matter what the exercises are, so long as they allow you to maintain your target heart rate. Of course, it's easier and more fun to perform such exercises to music. Put on your favorite rock CD and attend your own little aerobics class.

Swimming and Aqua-Jogging

Swimming is a wonderful exercise that uses most of your muscles without damaging them. But you may find it difficult to swim fast enough to maintain your target rate without tiring your arms. Be sure to wear your heart monitor and check your heart rate regularly. If you can't maintain your target rate, try a different exercise.

Simply treading water is a great way to use most of your muscles, and it is better suited than swimming to a strictly aerobic objective. You can perform such "aqua-jogging" with the help of a floatation vest that you can purchase in most sporting goods stores. Your upright position will make it easier for you to check the time, monitor your heart rate, and converse with friends. Any repetitive motion involving your arms and legs will suffice. Try aqua-jogging or aqua-treading, or aqua-cross-country skiing. You can vary your exercise every few minutes to keep any particular group of muscles from getting sore. You can also increase the water's resistance to make it easier to maintain your target heart rate by wearing sneakers or more clothing in the water.

There is one big drawback, however, to any exercise performed in water. Unless you are fortunate enough to have a pool, you cannot perform it at home. If exercise in water means using a public pool or gym, consider the extra time that transportation, changing, and showering require. You haven't found the right exercise if you're not willing and able to perform it every day.

Stretching

It is important to stretch your legs after any exercise that uses them on a daily basis, and if you are running or fast walking, you should stretch them before as well. This keeps them flexible and minimizes soreness and risk of injury. There are many stretches to choose from, but here is a sequence that works for me, and you can complete it in just a few minutes. For each of the following five stretches, count slowly to twenty. Don't stretch and loosen, stretch and loosen, or "bounce" your limbs, the way some people do. Instead, sustain a full, steady stretch for the entire count, while pushing gently to keep the relevant muscle at its stretching limit. Your maximum extension will increase somewhat over the course of your stretch, but don't stretch too hard. If you stretch the muscle to its limit, not beyond, greater flexibility will come with time.

1. Placing your hands against a wall or gripping something tall and stable (like a horizontal bar), kick your left leg straight out behind you, extending it fully. Now slowly lower your *right* knee forward and down in front of you. This will create a stretch of your *left* hind calf muscle. Keep your left foot flat on the ground, and be sure you feel the stretch at the back, top part of your calf.

2. Without straightening your right knee or moving your left foot, bend your *left* knee somewhat as well. This will create a stretch of the left *front* calf muscle. Be sure you feel the stretch at the *bottom* front of the calf.

Switching the roles of each leg, perform the same two stretches for the right calf muscles.

3. Holding something tall and stable with your right hand for balance, kick your left calf back behind you, grab your left ankle with your left hand, and pull your left foot back and up, so that its heel touches the middle of your left buttock. This will produce a stretch of your left front thigh muscle. Extend your left thigh backward behind you so that you're sure you feel the stretch in your left front thigh.

Do the same thing with your right leg to produce a stretch of your right front thigh muscle.

4. Kick your left leg out straight to your left side, extend it fully, and then bend your right knee outward and down to the right. Now, place both of your hands on your right knee, and slowly bend your right knee down further. This will produce a stretch of your left inner thigh muscle (your left hamstring). Be careful to maintain your balance. Once you have the idea of this stretch, place your hands on a tall and stable object (rather than on your right knee) and use it to support some of your weight while you lower your right knee.

Reverse the roles of your legs to perform the same stretch for your right hamstring.

5. Grabbing something tall and stable for balance, kick your left

leg straight out in front of you and rest the heel of your left foot on a coffee table, chair, or other convenient flat surface. Your left leg should extend out from your body at a 90-degree angle. Now slowly bend your right knee forward and down. This will produce a stretch of the muscle in the back of your left thigh. Adjust the stretch to be sure you feel the stretch there and not in the back of your left calf.

Reverse the roles of your legs to stretch the muscle in the back of your right thigh.

How Long Should I Exercise?

There is no clear answer, but studies suggest you should perform your exercise for at least thirty minutes. Moreover, you should exercise continuously. If you stop and rest, your heart rate will fall, and you'll have to spend additional exercise time just to bring it back up again. Also, if you stop, your body will realize that you *can* stop, and it will devote itself to persuading you to stop, rather than to getting rid of your excess fat deposits. In other words, even though it sounds easier to stop and rest, it actually isn't. The more you stop, the more your body will resist you. You'll never get in the habit of exercising for thirty minutes each day unless you learn to do so continuously. If you must stop for some specific reason—to adjust your exercise machine, change the channel on the television set, grab the phone, answer the doorbell, or pick up the pen you just dropped—jog in place, so your heart rate doesn't drop. If you feel you're just about to give in to temptation and stop, lower the level of your exercise, or slow down your pace, to bring your pulse down by about ten beats per minute. Believe it or not, this will feel as though you are taking a break. Raise the level back up to your target rate after you feel refreshed.

You may find that thirty minutes of continuous exercise is hard to accomplish at first. If so, try working your way up to it. Start out by doing half an hour each day with your heart rate at only 110. That's not high enough to keep you thin, but it will be high enough to get you started. You'll soon feel bored and ready to push yourself to 120. Before you know it, you'll be up to 130, and so on. One of the tricks that worked well for me when I first started was the "sprint finale." After I had finished thirty minutes at whatever rate I felt comfortable with, I would go all out for a minute or two to see what I could do. I knew I was free to stop at any time, because I had already finished my thirty minutes. But I was often surprised by how easy the sprint was. I sometimes even enjoyed it. That helped me realize my body could handle a higher exercise level. Next I would try a couple of minutes at the higher level during the middle of my exercise period, going back down to the lower level as soon as I felt taxed. Before I knew it, I was exercising at the higher level in general.

Here are two more tips for making your exercise easier.

First, exercise where it is cool. Exercise generates a lot of heat, and pumping blood to your skin to cool your body down is a lot of extra work for your heart. Exercising where it is cool improves your body's "attitude" toward your exercise. Your body may be resisting your exercise because it is getting too hot. Wouldn't you rather have your body be pushing *you* to exercise, the way it sometimes does on a cold winter day?

Also, be sure to dress lightly. If you are going to sweat, you might as well get the benefit. The purpose of sweat is to let the air cool you down by causing the sweat to evaporate. This can't happen if the air is blocked by a lot of clothing. One of the best ways to keep cool indoors is to use a fan. If you exercise at home, buy a large one and position it so that it blows directly on your back when you exercise. This accelerates the evaporation process. If there's a cool breeze outside, try opening the windows.

Second, provide yourself with a distraction.

A lot of people enjoy listening to music while they exercise. If you are not at home or otherwise can't turn a stereo on, a Walkman-type radio or tape player is cheap, light, and merciful to other people who would prefer not to hear your music. I especially recommend music with a beat, because it lets you feel like you are dancing or otherwise responding to it. Not only is this pleasurable, but it tends to make the exercise seem easier. Think of how easy it is to dance to rock music. This is, of course, part of the idea behind most aerobics classes.

Another alternative is to read a newspaper, a magazine, or a good book. Time flies when you are reading something interesting. Better yet, try marking up papers or doing similar work. I find the exercise bike best suited to this activity. Time also flies when you are absorbed in your work. You look up, thirty minutes have passed, and you have killed two birds with one stone.

Some people like listening to books on tape. Some enjoy watching television. Some people have a good time conversing with a family member or friend, and you can even use a portable phone for this purpose (with a headset, so you don't strain your neck). Conversation won't interfere with your exercise, and it makes the time pass quickly. But you may have to gulp some air between phrases when you speak, so use your exercise time to catch up with those friends and relatives who prefer to do most of the talking anyway.

If all else fails, try daydreaming. It's amazing how absorbing a daydream can be. By the time you've finished with your schemes and triumphs, the thirty minutes will have passed.

What Time of Day Should I Exercise?

I recommend exercising in the morning, just after you wake up, and before you have breakfast, for several reasons.

First, your exercise may seem easier on an empty stomach, because you won't have to divert blood from your stomach to perform it. Don't worry about not having enough energy. Your body has plenty of energy stored to meet your needs, and you'll feel fine once your exercise is under way.

Second, if you exercise before your morning shower, you won't have to shower a second time after your exercise. This will save you precious time. Don't forget, you're going to be doing this every day.

Third, early in the morning is the best time to perform outdoor exercises like jogging or fast walking. The temperature is still cool, and there are fewer cars to annoy you and impede your progress.

Fourth, your exercise will elevate your mood and your metabolism and make your whole day go better. You'll be missing out on this benefit if you exercise at night and then go to bed.

But the main reason to exercise first thing in the morning is that it is the easiest time of day to have an inviolable routine. You're never going to say to yourself, "Oh, darn, I got caught up in that meeting and missed my exercise routine" if your exercise routine takes place at 7:00 a.m. Neither are you going to say, "I know I'm supposed to exercise now, but I'm so exhausted, I just can't bear the thought of it." If you're serious about your exercise routine, you'll do it first thing in the morning so you can get it out of the way. If you are not serious, you'll put it off until the afternoon or evening, and then not get around to it at all.

How Often Should I Exercise?

The answer to this question is worth repeating:
Every single day.
"What was that you said? Five times per week?!"
No, I said every single day.
"Surely it's enough to exercise every other day. That's what all my friends do. That's what the people at the gym recommend."
Your friends are not trying to send their bodies a message, and the people at the gym think you are trying to burn off fat. You are not going to persuade your body that you *must* stay thin if whole days go by when you are completely sedentary. Your body will realize that your exercise is at your discretion and it can therefore

afford to store fat. It will respond by trying to discourage you from exercising. Studies have demonstrated that exercising only a few times a week won't keep you thin in the long run.

"Surely you don't mean that I have to exercise on vacation." Yes, I do. I said every single day.

"What if once in a blue moon I'm simply exhausted and can't bear the thought of exercise? Surely I can skip a day."

If you do that, the blue moon will come once a week, then twice a week, then three times a week, and you will not be thin.

"But that's an enormous commitment. How do you expect me to find the time?"

It's only thirty minutes. If you buy an exercise machine, walk fast, or jog, you won't have to go to the gym. If you exercise when you get up in the morning, you won't have to shower twice. There's no need to turn this into a major hassle. Protracted regimes consisting of drives to the gym, changes of clothing, warmups, extra showers, conversations with friends, and so forth, that serve to turn a half-hour activity into a two-hour affair are merely forms of procrastination.

"But my life is crazed with children, work, and other commitments from morning till night. How do you expect me to fit in a daily exercise regime?"

Do you ever sleep? Good. Set your clock so that it wakes you up thirty minutes sooner than you would otherwise rise. As soon as you wake up, perform your exercise routine in your room, or in another room if your spouse or companion is asleep, and don't tell anyone else you are awake. If you are fast walking or jogging, slip quietly out the door. Then start your hectic, crazy, nonstop, can't-find-the-time day.

"But I'm often at meetings or on vacation in remote places where there are no exercise machines."

Learn to jog or walk fast as a backup. If it's cold or raining outside, try jogging back and forth down a hallway or around a large room; or try performing stepping exercises to music.

"I sometimes take a vacation hiking or bicycling in the mountains. Do I have to do my exercise then as well?"

If that is how you are spending your vacation, it should be fairly easy to get in half an hour a day of aerobic exercise. But I concede that the one time you do not need to perform your daily exercise is when you are already spending *most* of your day engaged in athletic activity. After all, you don't need to persuade your body that you are active if you really are. In such a case, you may want to save your legs for your principal vacation activity. Be careful not to kid yourself, though. Spending the whole day hiking, or rock climbing, or bicycling, or playing tennis qualifies. Spending the day gardening or playing golf does not. Similarly, if you are about to play two hours of competitive tennis without stopping, and you are sure that your heart rate will remain elevated throughout, perhaps you can skip your normal exercise. But casual stop-and-go tennis, football, or basketball does not qualify.

"What if I'm sick?"

That's an exception. Don't exercise if you're sick. Listen to your body. It will let you know if you're still too sick to exercise.

"I don't mind a little exercise, but let's not go crazy. Surely it's not worth all this effort."

How much effort are we talking about? Once you get this thirty minutes out of the way, you won't have to be active again all day. You can spend the rest of the day lounging about in an easy chair. What's more, you will be able to eat whatever you want. Is staying thin, looking good, and feeling great while eating whatever you want worth thirty minutes a day to you? If not, that's fine, but then don't expect to stay thin by dieting. Daily exercise is far less trouble and effort than dieting, and far more effective.

When Can I Stop Performing This Daily Exercise Routine?

The answer is, *never*. As I explained in chapter 1, Lamarck's hypothesis has been proven wrong. Exercise will change your body, but it will not change your genes. Your genetic inheritance will always say, "While active, keep thin; while sedentary, store fat." If you become sedentary again, your marvelously flexible biology will respond by reintroducing vital fat stores, and I don't mean eventually. I mean within a few weeks. Don't forget our discussion in chapter 2. When you become sedentary, your body says to itself, "Aha, either winter has arrived, and there is no food around to be gathered, or I am injured and can't reach food sources. Time to turn myself into a human refrigerator." Pick an exercise you enjoy and that you think you can sustain for the rest of your life, for your body is like Cinderella's coach. As soon as you stop exercising, it will turn back into a pumpkin.

"Then what's the point? At least if I go on a diet, I keep the weight off."

No, you don't. Think what happened the last time you went on a diet. Didn't you put all the weight back on as soon as you stopped dieting?

"Then why is exercise any better than dieting?"

There are many good reasons. We discussed some of them in Chapter 1, and we discuss more of them in the next chapter. But the most important reason is that you can't stay on a diet for the rest of your life, and you wouldn't want to. You can't spend the rest of your life fighting with your body about what your weight should be. It would be a miserable, food-obsessed, sluggish, depressed, and frustrating existence, but more important, your body would win in the end. A normal-weight person like you cannot win a long-term battle with your body over how much fat it should be storing.

But you *can* maintain a thirty-minute daily exercise regime for the rest of your life, and if you do, you *will* stay thin for the rest of your life. What's more, the life you live will be happier, healthier, stronger, more energetic, and more fun.

Disclaimer

Before we conclude this chapter, it's time for an important disclaimer. If you peruse any exercise book, you'll notice that it keeps telling you, "Take it easy." There's a good reason for this. The author and the publisher are legally liable if they tell you otherwise. Suppose, for example, that millions of people were to read this book and follow its advice. There would likely be a few who should not be exercising at all given their delicate physical conditions. There would also be a few who could exercise mildly—a relaxed stroll in the park—but who would be ill advised to maintain substantially elevated heart rates for extended periods. Some of these people could even have heart attacks or strokes if they performed aerobic exercise. While one would normally expect such people to know who they are, there might still be a few of them who can't, or don't, listen to their bodies, and who, after reading this book, will exercise even though they shouldn't.

Now it's a funny thing about our society, but if such people were to read this book and then suffer a heart attack or stroke, they could, and probably *would*, sue me for advocating exercise. If they actually died, their estates would be glad to sue instead. Unless I make it very clear to such people that they should *not* be exercising, I could be legally liable for the dire consequences of their 'decision to exercise. Unfortunately, if all the rest of us limit our exercise to the pace that such unusually frail people can withstand, then all the rest of us will be chubby. As a legal matter, therefore, I'm actually not permitted to tell you how to stay thin, on account of my legal liability for the unlikely circumstance that you should not be trying to.

So here it is—my warning—and please pay close attention, because I am very serious about it, notwithstanding my sarcasm:

You are following my advice about how to stay thin at your own risk. There are some people who could *die* from exercising, and you could be one of them. This book has been written for *healthy* people. I know nothing about your particular physical condition. But even if you are healthy, I do not know, and cannot know, the heart rate that it would be best for you to maintain while exercising, and even if I did, I am not a doctor, and I have not been trained to give medical advice. You should therefore consult your private physician before instituting a regime of daily aerobic exercise and deciding what your target heart rate should be. You obviously should not be performing aerobic exercise if you are elderly or in poor health, or have any sort of condition that might make aerobic exercise unsafe. Even if you are healthy, young, and unconcerned, however, you must bear the following in mind: I take absolutely no responsibility for the potentially lethal consequences of your deciding to exercise, at *any* pace. I know what the right pace of exercise is for me, but I have no idea what the right pace of exercise is for you.

4.

Jack Sprat Was on Pritikin; His Wife Was on Atkins

FOR AS LONG AS YOU HAVE BEEN LEADING a sedentary existence, you have been trying to force your body to store less fat than it has wanted to store. You therefore could not trust your body to keep you as thin as you wanted to be. To the contrary, your body was a traitor, trying to undermine your efforts to stay thin by persuading you to eat enough to let it restore its fat deposits. But you lacked the equipment required to know how much to eat on your own. A variation of as little as 100 calories per day could cause you to gain ten pounds per year. You couldn't possibly calculate your caloric intake with enough precision to maintain your physical form. Your body has evolved complex feedback loops that allow it to maintain its levels of fat over time. Without the help of those mechanisms, you were lost in a food wilderness. "To eat, or not to eat?" you asked yourself at every turn, and every answer seemed arbitrary.

"Should I stop eating this sandwich now? I've already eaten half of it. Is that enough, or will I be hungry again soon? I *want* to eat the second half, but I'll be that much thinner if I can manage not to eat it. Come to think of it, I probably shouldn't have eaten the first half. I probably could have gotten away with eating no sandwich at all. How about if I don't eat the second half, but I *do* have just a few of these French fries? Surely a few wouldn't hurt, and just a few French fries must have fewer calories than the second half of this sandwich. But what if I start eating them and find I can't stop? What if I wind up eating them all? It has happened before. Come to think of it, it seems that I've already eaten the second half of this sandwich, and most of the French fries as well."

You likewise couldn't rely on your body to tell you *what* to eat. Your body would only have led you to binge on high-calorie sugars and fats. For guidance, you therefore turned to whatever diet book you had been reading of late, along with its accompanying calorie- or carbohydrate-counting tables, meal plans, recipes, and inviolable prescriptions. The resulting behavior was artificial, to say the least.

"I shouldn't be eating the bread on this sandwich. I'll scrape out the middle of the sandwich with my teeth, the way you do with an Oreo, and leave the bread on the plate. I hope no one notices. Oh, darn. I was being so good, but now it seems as though I've eaten most of the bread as well. But I couldn't help myself—it was so delicious. I should have just eaten the whole sandwich to begin with."

"I shouldn't be eating the fatty meat in this sandwich. Maybe I can pull the fat off and just eat the lean. Maybe I can pull the meat out, and just eat the bread. Maybe I should pull out the tomatoes. I think they were on the 'bad list.' I wonder if I could wipe off some of this mayonnaise. Maybe I can do it discreetly with a piece of the turkey. But where should I wipe it? On the side of the plate? Someone might notice. What if I wipe it under the table, like chewing gum?"

"Am I supposed to be eating these beets? One part of my diet book said I should be, but another part of it said I shouldn't be. One book had them on the 'must eat' list, but another book had them on the 'never eat' list. One book said I could only eat them raw, but another book said I could only eat them cooked. I think I'm allowed to eat them raw before dinner, but I have to eat them cooked during dinner; or is it the other way around? I think I'm allowed to eat them in combination with leafy greens, but not in combination with tomatoes or peppers. I think I can eat them, but if I do, it's essential that I not eat celery the following day."

This endless circle of obsessions and inquiries, divorced from any physical sensation—divorced, in fact, from any physical reality—invariably led to the following kinds of recriminations: "Why did I eat all that? That was practically a binge. I ate the entire bowl of cashews. I ate the whole bag of potato chips. I had a third helping of the pasta, and nobody else even had seconds. I had a bottle of wine, a large salad full of cheese and oil, a big helping of pâté with toast points, an enormous fatty steak, a giant baked potato loaded with butter and sour cream, creamed spinach, broccoli hollandaise, three dinner rolls with butter, a large piece of banana cream pie, two cherry cordials, five petits-fours—and I'm still eating!"

Is this any surprise? What, after all, is there to make you *stop* eating? If fullness were a sign in the road, it would be a very small sign covered up by a thicket, and you would be driving past it at eighty miles per hour, caught up in an internal monologue. Why should you even be looking for signs of "fullness"? You don't heed your body when it tells you to start eating. You don't heed your body when it tells you *what* to eat. You don't heed your body when it tells you to *keep* eating. Why should you heed it when it tells you to stop?

But now that you are exercising every day—now that you and your body agree that you should not be storing fat—you can allow your *body* to decide when you should be eating and when you should stop. You can keep on eating that sandwich until you feel full and know you are doing the right thing. "I'm always hungry, and I'm never full," I can hear you saying. "If I eat whenever I want to, I'll wind up fat as a pig." But that's only because, until now, you have been too sedentary. You really *were* hungry all the time, even when you were full, because your body was trying to store more fat. Now that you are exercising every day, your body will make you lose interest in food. Your body will even secrete chemicals, like leptin, that will keep you from maintaining higher fat levels by making you feel satiated when your stomach is empty. Until now you have been assuming that your mind controls your body and tells it when to eat. But the truth is precisely the opposite. Your body controls your mind with chemicals and feedback loops that tell *you* when to eat and when to stop. Studies show that people who exercise stay thin in the long run without *trying* to eat less. You don't believe me? Keep up your daily exercise up for just a few months and see what I mean.

You likewise can, and should, let your body tell you *what* to eat. You should prepare or order the foods that seem most appetizing to you and eat the food on your plate that tastes the best. Studies show that people who exercise stay thin in the long run regardless of what they eat, and neither a high-fat diet nor a high-carbohydrate diet makes them gain weight. Besides, your body is not going to crave meals consisting of nothing but sugars and fats. Your body will direct your appetite and sense of taste to obtain the foods *it* needs to maintain its health and form. When eight-month-old babies were allowed to choose among different kinds of food, they all ate balanced diets, and some even cured themselves of rickets by eating large quantities of cod liver oil. Do you think you can perform as well as those babies?

You've probably already noticed that balanced meals taste best. Steak is delicious, but after some number of bites, the potatoes taste even better, and you turn to eating them. Meat is fine on its own, and bread is fine on its own, but they taste best together in a hamburger or a sandwich. Similarly, variation tastes best. You may have a craving for fried chicken, and when you finally have it for dinner, it tastes as delicious as you had imagined. But if you have it for dinner again the next night, it doesn't taste as good. This is no accident. Your body *wants* you to eat a balanced diet. If you exercise daily, you will crave meat, vegetables, salads, fruits, bread, eggs, cheese, and potatoes, because your body needs them to maintain its physical form. Any effort you make to avoid certain kinds of food will be counterproductive, because it will interfere with your body's efforts. It will continue a pattern in which you ignore your body's signals and substitute decisions based on internal dialectics that have nothing to do with your body's needs.

That is what is so frustrating about most diet books. Their authors insist that you avoid certain foods, but doing so becomes increasingly difficult and unpleasant as your body fights to get you to eat the foods it needs. According to some of these authors, human beings were not designed to eat many of the things that are available in modern society. But does this make any sense? You've taken basic biology. Do you think that millions of years of evolution have left your body unprepared to deal with a foodstuff like bread? Do you think your body can be defeated by encounters with corn, rice, sugar, potatoes, butter, fat, or oil? Human beings are omnivores, and they were pretty much designed to eat everything but grass and leaves. If it smells and tastes good to you, then you were designed to eat it. If you have eaten too much of it, you will lose your appetite for it.

According to other authors, it is not the mere presence of these foods that human beings were not prepared for, but rather their abundance. Left to their natural impulses, human beings will keep on eating these foods until they get fat. Does this make any more sense? When hunters and gatherers found food in prehistoric times, did they go on devouring it until they became fat, and bring nothing home to their families? If this were true, there wouldn't be any thin people around today. Teenagers and college athletes would be as fat as their sedentary, middle-aged parents. After all, no one has been depriving teenagers of food. Do they have more self-restraint than their parents have?

The reason you are storing more fat than you'd like is not because certain foods weren't meant to be eaten. It is because your body *wants* to store more fat. These are *good* foods that make it easy for your body to maintain the form it wants to maintain. If you exercise every day, your body uses these foods to maintain a thin and athletic form, rather than to store fat. But if you remain sedentary, choosing certain foods will not keep your body from storing more fat in the long run. It will only make your life less pleasant. So stop removing the fat, the skin, the breading, the sauce, the butter, or the sugar from your food, unless you are doing so for medical reasons unrelated to your weight. To the extent that such behavior lowers the caloric content of your food, you will just wind up eating more food to maintain yourself. It is not more fun to eat fifty bites of diet food than it is to eat thirty bites of regular food. The point of eating is to wind up feeling satisfied.

Besides, these authors all contradict each other. According to one group, you must avoid fat and oil and live primarily on bread, rice, pasta, cereal, potatoes (with no butter), and other carbohydrates. According to another group, however, you must avoid bread, rice, pasta, cereal, potatoes, and other carbohydrates and live primarily on fatty meat and cheese. According to a third group, you must avoid simple carbohydrates, like those found in bread, potatoes, rice, and pasta, and live primarily on meat and complex carbohydrates, like those found in whole-grain cereals and fruits. According to a fourth group, you must also avoid meat and live solely on complex carbohydrates and fiber. According to a fifth group, you must carefully measure and combine proteins, carbohydrates, and fats in a magical proportion that your incompetent body is incapable of maintaining on its own.

The much-publicized positions of these opposing diet camps make for entertaining reading in newspapers and magazines, and I suppose one can say in their collective favor that, like Jack Sprat and his wife, their adherents shall together lick the platter clean. But that is little consolation to the person who is trying to stay thin. What could be more frustrating, after months of self-deprivation, than to open your newspaper and read that your diet is a fraud and you should in fact have been doing precisely the opposite?

Many of these authors also insist that the food you eat be low in calories or eaten in very small quantities, so that the unfortunate dieter consumes fewer than 1,500 calories per day. For some reason, the other members of the species are capable of consuming twice as much while staying thin as rails. But readers of these books are told that they are the biologically "chosen." They alone must eat like birds; this is their special cross to bear. Fortunately, multimillion-dollar industries are standing by with frozen dinners that are low in calories and high in price, packaged together with the author's blessing.

Some authors also have special rules about *when* you can eat. Some advise you to eat many small meals throughout the day. Some advise you to alternate gorging with fasting. Some insist that you eat your entire meal within sixty minutes. Some advise you to alternate low-carbohydrate meals with high-carbohydrate meals, or meat meals with vegetarian meals.

Regardless of whether they focus on what, how much, or when you can eat, all these diets become increasingly unpleasant, and increasingly difficult to follow, over time. Moreover, they seem to work less and less well, as if the body were somehow catching on to them. With each minor, but inevitable, transgression, much of the lost weight seems to come back. You can buy diet books by the armful and try to figure out which of their assertions are right, or at least which of them are right for you. But before you do, you should ask yourself whether *any* of them is right for you. The fact that you see a man or woman in a white coat on a diet book's cover should not lead you to assume that the book's assertions are supported by objective evidence. If there were conclusive proof to support the book's assertions, the diet controversy would be over. Nor should you be swayed by the book's claim that its assertions are corroborated by the experiences of hundreds of people. It is really not possible to prove claims of this sort. Too many other variables affect human behavior and human weight, and it is not possible to establish adequate controls. The assertions made in diet books differ in this regard from refutable medical assertions, such as that a particular disease is caused by a particular virus, or that a particular vaccine prevents a particular disease.

But one thing you can know for sure is that these diet books can't all be right. In fact, since they all contradict each other, you are logically forced to conclude that most of them are wrong.

When objective knowledge is not available and purported experts all disagree with each other, the things you accept as true should at least make sense to you and be consistent with your own experience. Suppose you were sick and your doctor told you to bleed out a quart of blood and then go running in the field. Suppose your doctor insisted, moreover, that many of his patients had followed his advice and been cured. You might well reason as follows: "First, this doctor's assertions seem counterintuitive. If my body needed less blood, it would surely have learned how to get rid of the excess without forcing me to cut myself open and possibly infect myself. It seems to have learned how to accomplish far more impressive things. Besides, I feel very tired, and my body apparently wants me to lie down and sleep. True, the doctor claims that many of his patients have been cured by his methods, but how do I know that they would not have gotten well without his advice? True, the doctor is a well-known and highly respected authority, but all these authorities seem to disagree with each other, and none of them has yet devised experiments that serve to prove their assertions." Suppose a second doctor then came to visit you, and her advice was to lie down and rest. At least that advice would seem consistent with your own common sense and experience. Wouldn't that be an argument in its favor?

In one sense, the mechanical sense, all diets "work," for they are all ways of depriving your body of the food it needs to maintain its form. You can accomplish this by simply not eating—in other words, by fasting. You can accomplish this more gradually by refusing to supply your body with enough food to match your daily caloric expenditures. As a more sophisticated alternative, you can selectively deprive your body of carbohydrates, so that it lacks the means to store fat. But your body is not going to respond to any of these mechanical solutions in the way you want it to. It is not going to say, "My, that's a clever approach; I guess I'll just give up trying to store fat." It follows that none of these diets is going to work for you in the long run. While you can use any of them to lose that extra twenty pounds of fat, you can never expect the weight to stay off when the diet is over.

Remember that your body doesn't think of that twenty pounds as extra fat. It thinks of it as vital tissue to be restored as soon as possible. This means that if you really want to use one of these diets to *stay* thin, you are going to have to stay on it for the rest of your life, and you are going to have to adhere to it religiously. You are going to have to perpetually maintain your body on the edge of starvation. Some people do this, and do it successfully, but it is a depressing, frustrating, and unpleasant existence.

I also recognize that there are some people whom exercise alone will not help. There are people whose bodies contain unusually large amounts of fat because they are suffering from what amounts to a disease, just as there are people who have difficulty maintaining normal sugar levels in their bloodstream because they have diabetes. Because of faulty genes, these people may secrete too much insulin, or have congenitally inactive thyroid glands, or experience other biological malfunctioning. There are also people who store unusually large amounts of fat for strictly psychological reasons. Certain diets may help some of these people.

As I explained in the introduction, however, this book is for the much larger group of people who are within a weight range that society considers normal but who are nevertheless storing a lot of fat (especially compared to what they used to store) and are not happy about it. In other words, this book is for someone like you. You wouldn't read a book that was written for someone with diabetes and follow its advice, expecting its recommendations to help you maintain your body's sugar levels. Why, then, would you read a book that was written for someone with abnormal weight problems and expect its recommendations to apply to you? What you want is to stay thin and toned, the way you were when you were twenty, on a permanent basis. A diet book is not going to help you accomplish this.

What about diet plus exercise? While most diet books do advocate exercise, they recommend it as an ancillary activity, from a passive, mechanical point of view. Their idea is that since daily weight gain or loss is based on the difference between caloric intake and caloric expenditure, you can lose weight not merely by decreasing the former but by increasing the latter. They therefore make such assertions as, "If you exercise for half an hour each day, you will burn an extra 300 calories per day; this may not sound like much, but over the course of a year, it adds up to thirty pounds." Are they implying that if you exercise for half an hour every day for a year, you will in fact lose thirty pounds? Are they further implying that if you keep on exercising, you will continue to lose thirty pounds per year until you die of starvation? I don't think the authors of most diet books spend much time reflecting on such questions. Yet common sense tells you that if you exercise, you *must* eat more to make up for the additional caloric expenditure. How much more you eat, and how much thinner you will therefore remain, will depend on what new weight your body wants to maintain. In other words, the question is not, "How many calories am I consuming or expending?" It is, "What is my new equilibrium?"

Because exercise obviously does lead the body to maintain a lower fat equilibrium, the exercise recommended by most diet books is effective to some extent. But because most people perform this exercise for the wrong reasons, the exercise rarely produces the right results. People do not exercise often enough, long enough, strenuously enough, or consistently enough to stay thin, and then they stop, because they cannot relate the exercise to any change in their weight. Even if they do become thinner for a while, they attribute the weight loss to the diet, rather than to the exercise. What they need to do is give up the diet and keep on exercising.

A lot of people stand to profit from your belief that dieting can keep you as thin as you want to be. Diet food is a hundred-billion-dollar industry. But the truth is that dieting will not make you thin, because the excess fat you've put on is *normal* for a sedentary person. If you are healthy, your body is not going to let you become *abnormal*. Unlike dieting, daily exercise lets you stay thin in the long run, because it is normal for an active person to be thin. Daily exercise lets you be just like the people you've been envying for so long: the people who seem to eat whatever they want to yet stay thin and toned; the people who are busy with business, and sports, and children, and activities, and for whom food seems to be the last thing on their minds. You are *not* permanently separated from those people by biological forces.

5.

Eat When You're Hungry; Stop When You're Full

IF UNTIL NOW YOU HAVE BEEN LIVING a sedentary life and fighting your body's resulting efforts to store fat, then you are probably out of touch with your body's natural sensations of hunger and satiety. Now that you are exercising every day and your body is your ally, you must learn to follow its commands. You must listen to your body when it tells you to stop eating and when it tells you to start eating again.

The sensation of fullness is hard to miss if you're looking for it, but it is also easy to bypass if you're not. Your unstretched stomach holds only about a quart of food. But your stomach is elastic, and it can stretch to hold much more. If you keep eating, there is, of course, a point at which your stomach has been stretched to its maximum capacity. Then you will receive clear signals of physical distress if you try to put any more food into it, and you will presumably leave the table announcing that you are "stuffed." But if this happens to you once a year at Thanksgiving, it is probably too often. You should get into the habit of watching for, and heeding, your body's signals of satiety.

I am reminded of a disgusting but funny scene from the Monty Python movie *The Meaning of Life*. In the middle of a fashionable restaurant, a man is sitting alone at a table, shoveling huge quantities of food into his mouth. After he has eaten all he can, a waiter appears.

"Would you care for a mint?" the waiter asks innocently.

"No, thanks," the man replies. "I'm *stuffed*."

"Oh, do go ahead," the waiter entreats. "They're wafer-thin."

"Oh, all right," the man replies, takes the mint, and eats it. As soon as he does, he explodes, and his innards cover the room.

There is actually a reason to stop when you are full, even though you are thin. Fullness is the point at which food stops tasting good. You've probably noticed this when you've gone ahead and had seconds of some delicious food that was being served for lunch or dinner, only to discover the second experience was not as pleasurable as the first. If you eat past the point of fullness, it's going to be that much longer before you are hungry and can really enjoy eating again. Thus, even if you are a complete hedonist whose principal objective is to maximize your eating pleasure (and I don't mind telling you that I certainly am), it is in your interest to recognize when you are full and stop eating at that point, so that you can look forward to your next meal (which, after all, is not very far off).

Okay, so how *do* you feel when you're full? Well, you feel the way you would if you had a gas tank inside of you. When you first start eating, the "tank" is empty, and the sensation of pressure from the introduction of food is at the bottom of the tank, the part that is receiving the food. As the food approaches the top of the rim, you start to feel pressure toward the top of the tank. When you are full, you feel pressure at the very top. The resulting sensation of fullness is accompanied by other signals of satiety. Your interest in the food on your plate decreases, and the food looks less appetizing. Your arm seems less eager to raise the food to your lips. Your mouth seems less interested in taking the food in and chewing it. As I mentioned, the food itself doesn't taste as good. There is a shift in the whole relationship between your mind and the food that is sitting in front of you. If you were a child, you would probably be turning to your parents at this point and saying, "May I be excused to go play now?"

One reason some people don't stop eating when they are full is that they don't want to waste what is left on their plates. They therefore allow an *external* cue (the point at which their plates are clean), rather than an *internal* cue (the point at which their stomachs are full), to determine when they stop eating. But this is not rational behavior. Suppose, for example, that you just spent $20 on a restaurant steak only to discover that you feel full after eating just half of it. The other $10 is wasted whether you eat the second half or not. The second half is not going to taste good, and it is not going to help either you or your body meet your respective objectives. If you've already made the mistake of buying more food than you can eat, why compound the problem by actually *eating* it? If you wish, ask the waiter to wrap the extra food so you can take it home in a doggy bag. I realize there are many troubling aspects to the world we live in, and maybe next time you would prefer to donate that $20 to UNICEF. But you will not help anyone else in the world by eating too much food.

Another reason many people don't stop when they are full is that fullness usually arrives before dessert. Desserts were designed for people to eat when they were already full. The normal solution is to have just a bite of dessert, preferably someone else's. But if you want to enjoy your own dessert, you must do what your mother told you to do when you were a child: "Save room for dessert!" When your mother said that, she didn't mean you should avoid packing so much into your belly that you literally couldn't stuff in dessert without exploding like the man in the Monty Python film. She meant you should stop while your stomach was still partly empty, so that eating dessert would only make it full. Remember that she was also the one who kept warning you not to *spoil* your appetite for dinner. She assumed that if you were full when dinner arrived, you wouldn't want to eat any of it.

But saving room for dessert is harder to do than it sounds, especially when the main course is delicious. Fullness comes on suddenly, and you have to know your body well to prevent it from happening. Besides, who knows whether dessert will even taste good? I therefore usually go for the gusto while I can and only sample the dessert when it arrives. Most of the time, it doesn't taste nearly as good as everyone claims. If I find myself feeling cheated out of my fair share of ice cream and cake, I sometimes do something unusual when I am eating alone: I *start* my meal with a dessert that I have been craving. I might, for example, start dinner with a hot fudge sundae and then continue on to the fried chicken. Naturally I feel full and have to stop after only one or two pieces of chicken, but I'm perfectly happy. I've had my cake and eaten it too. If I did it the usual way, I wouldn't be able to resist eating three or four pieces of chicken, and then I would be too full to eat the sundae.

Having said all this, let me caution you not to err in the other direction. Don't stop eating before you are full, and don't try to persuade yourself that you are full if you aren't. Your body won't be fooled into keeping you thinner if you refuse to sate its appetite. You will just wind up eating more later on. There are some diet books that exhort you to eat lots of small meals throughout the day. I don't know what this accomplishes other than to make you more obsessed with food and less of a normal person. By the time you're done preparing and clearing up all those meals, how much time will you have left for life's other tasks? The sensation of fullness is one of life's pleasures, and there is nothing to be gained by denying it to yourself.

Likewise, don't try to fool your body by filling your stomach up with diet food. It's futile to eat nothing but salad with low-calorie dressing, or meat with no carbohydrates, and then search for signs of fullness. You have doubtless experienced the sense in which you are full but not satisfied when you indulge in such behavior. Your body is aware of the fact that it has not yet obtained the food it needs to maintain its physical form. You walk away from the table still thinking about food, and you wind up eating more later on. Doing such things is counterproductive, because they make it impossible for you and your body to cooperate to maintain your form. You will not learn to recognize and follow your body's signal of fullness if it keeps turning out to be a false signal that is not accompanied by satiety and does not accomplish the result that your body desires. Your objective is to make yourself thin for the rest of your life, not to make yourself thin for the next day and a half. Don't sabotage the process.

Let's move on to eating when you are hungry. What I really mean is, don't eat when you're not hungry. I recognize that life offers many opportunities to eat between meals. I realize we sometimes eat strictly for entertainment (going out for ice cream, for example), and we sometimes eat to put off doing undesirable work. But if you are performing your daily exercise, you will have little desire to eat between meals, and you should generally avoid doing so. Listen to your body when you are offered a snack and utter the polite "No, thank you" that the circumstances warrant. If your objectives are oral stimulation, entertainment, or procrastination, have some coffee, tea, or gum.

The bigger tactical problem is what to do when you are not hungry yet but mealtime has arrived. It is your lunch hour, your *only* lunch hour; or dinner is being served; or everyone is going out to eat *now*. Obviously you need to use your judgment, and this means you should consider how long it has been since your last meal and how much you ate at it. If, based on these facts, you're pretty sure you're going to be hungry soon, then go ahead and eat. Your body will adjust and pick up your appetite for you. One thing I've noticed is, just as they say "The darkest hour is right before the dawn," the fullest hour is right before you're hungry. The reason is that your stomach is busy clearing out your last meal and making room for your next. If it has been five hours since your last meal and you feel not the slightest bit hungry (or even feel surprisingly full), but all sorts of noise and commotion are going on in your digestive tract, then you can expect to be ravenous within the hour. So don't rush to declare that you aren't hungry and wind up eating crow.

In any case, it helps to plan your life so that your meals tend to occur when you are normally hungry. If you keep finding, for example, that dinner is served before you are hungry, see what you can do to arrange a later dinner hour, or an earlier lunch hour. If on weekdays you normally have a bowl of cereal for breakfast, plan to have lunch at noon. But if one day you have an unusually large breakfast, plan to have lunch at two. If on weekends you enjoy an enormous breakfast of bacon, eggs, potatoes, and pancakes, plan to skip lunch altogether and eat an early dinner. Common sense will tell you what plans to make so that you are likely to be eating again when you are hungry.

Don't be afraid to skip a meal if you really aren't hungry. Suppressing your appetite is one of the ways in which your body maintains your weight. If your levels of stored fat get too high, your body secretes leptin and other chemicals that make you feel satiated even though your stomach is empty. But don't err in the other direction. *Do* eat when you *are* hungry, and don't keep putting your hunger off, based on the misconception that doing so will somehow make you thinner. You can't fool your body into keeping you thinner by skipping meals. And if you don't listen to your body when it tells you to eat, you're not going to be able to listen to it when it tells you to stop.

Moreover, while we have all experienced the gnawing hunger pains which demand that we eat immediately, they are rare in adult life. The body recognizes that adults often have important tasks that they must finish before they pause to eat. Adult hunger therefore usually takes the form of a heightened sensation of appetite coupled with a moderate sensation of emptiness. It also tends to be a polite visitor. If it knocks and you are occupied, it goes away and does not come back for a while. So try to take note of the signs of your own hunger. Notice if your appetite seems to have picked up and food is crossing your mind, or if there is no longer any sense of satiety in your stomach. Ask yourself how long it has been since you last ate. If you're not sure whether you're hungry or not, try putting a piece of food in your mouth to see how your mouth responds to it. If your throat practically gulps the food down, you're hungry, and if it responds with indifference, you're not.

As for what to eat, we already discussed that in chapter 4: Eat balanced and varied meals consisting of the foods that appeal to you and that taste good. Millions of years of evolution have adequately equipped your body to know what foods it needs to maintain your physical form. Eating the foods you like is one of life's greatest pleasures. As the Bible says, it is your portion under the sun. If it is French fries you love, then order and enjoy them. You accomplish nothing by denying them to yourself. Just be sure to eat them only when you are hungry and to stop eating them when you are full.

I will concede that there is one form of food that evolution did not entirely prepare us for: alcoholic drinks. Drinks do not serve to make you full, so there is no natural limit to your capacity to imbibe them. I'd gladly tell you never to drink again, but then I'd have to follow my own advice. I'm reminded of St. Augustine's famous prayer: "Lord, make me chaste—but not yet." What I *am* going to suggest is that you drink in moderation.

I have two specific suggestions in this regard. First, treat drinks like food. That means, don't drink until you're hungry. Don't drink in the middle of the afternoon, for example, even though you are lying out by the pool and a sea breeze or daiquiri would be the perfect thing. Likewise, don't drink when you're full. Don't get in the habit of drinking cordials after dinner, for example.

Second, don't get drunk. There is an analogy here to the distinction between being full and being stuffed. If you are drinking on an empty stomach, one cocktail should be enough to give you a pleasant buzz. There is no need to have a second. Similarly, have *one* margarita before you enjoy dinner at your favorite Mexican restaurant, *not* margaritas throughout. Beer and wine, of course, are meant to be imbibed with food. But two glasses of either should be enough.

Don't get drunk just because you're at a party. If you feel the need for a prop, you can always sip club soda with lime. Getting drunk diminishes your capacity to be witty and charming, to make new friends and acquaintances, and to connect with old ones and find out how they are doing. If you're single, getting drunk diminishes, rather than increases, your chances of meeting and connecting with someone. In other words, getting drunk undermines everything you were trying to accomplish by coming to the party. And then you face the problem of how to get home safely.

6.

Stop Obsessing About Your Weight

Now that you're exercising every day, you can stop monitoring your weight. Your objective is to let your body maintain your weight without getting in its way. You have to learn to trust that your body really is keeping you thin. This is partly a matter of changing your psychological habits. Here are a few suggestions.

Avoid the Scale and the Mirror

Diets are unpleasant, and you wouldn't want to stay on one for long. You basically say to yourself, "I had better lose that ten pounds in four weeks, or I'm going to be very unhappy. I certainly won't be able to maintain my willpower if I don't see that I'm making progress." (Never mind the fact that you are going to gain the weight back as soon the diet is over. Hope springs eternal.) You therefore ask yourself every day, or even every hour, "How much progress am I making? Is staying on this diet worth the privation I'm putting up with?" You're never really sure, and you certainly don't want to deprive yourself for nothing. So you get on the scale every morning, and sometimes several times a day, to see how you are doing.

If your weight has gone down, you are of course relieved. Even if it has gone down only a little bit, at least you are getting somewhere.

If your weight has stayed the same, you're depressed. Maybe you really are wasting your time. If your weight has gone up, you are really upset. How could this have happened when you've been so good? Could it have been that little slip you made at your friend's house, when you nibbled a few of those cashews she set down in front of you? That friend is so inconsiderate. You invariably try other scales, to see if you can do better. It's a little like getting a second opinion. There's the scale in the bathroom at your friend's house. She won't know if you pretend to be going to the bathroom, then slip off your shoes and check your weight. There's that old scale packed away in the closet upstairs. Maybe it's time to pull it out and give it a shot. Maybe the time has come to buy a new scale altogether. You could splurge and buy one of those expensive scales

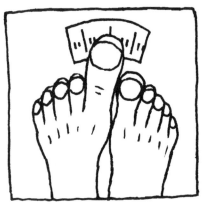

they sell in the department store. All too often, though, the other scales confirm the first scale's unwelcome diagnosis: your diet isn't working anymore.

When you're not checking out the scale, you're checking out your body. You're pinching your fat deposits to see how thick they feel. You're looking

at your bulges in the mirror to see if they look bigger or smaller. You're trying to figure out how fat your face is, or how much space there is between your thighs. Some days you like what you see. You're pretty sure you're getting somewhere. Other days, it's obvious to you that you're fat, hopelessly fat, fat and worthless.

All this behavior is not merely counterproductive. It's illogical. Much of the variation you observe from day to day in your weight *or* your appearance is attributable to water bloat. Your weight can vary by as much as ten pounds on account of changes in the amount of water in your body. Some baseball pitchers lose more than ten pounds when they pitch a game. Wrestlers, boxers, and jockeys do this intentionally (by sweating, and by other means that are not worth mentioning) before they are weighed for a match or race. Water bloat looks exactly like real fat in the mirror. It increases the size of all your fat bulges. One reason you look worst when you get up in the morning is that you have been lying flat all night, and the water in your body has drifted back into your face. Water bloat makes your eyes look smaller and your face less angular. There is therefore no way to know how much fat you have gained or lost on a day-by-day basis.

Your weight also varies with the amount of sugar stored in your muscles as a temporary energy source. This glycogen is packed with water, and its weight can vary by as much as five pounds. You store less glycogen in your muscles when you stop eating carbohydrates. But the resulting weight loss is temporary and reverses as soon as you start eating carbohydrates again. Naturally, your weight also varies with the amount of food in your stomach. You put on several pounds of weight when you eat your dinner.

Dieting tends to lower all these temporary weight variables. It results in temporary dehydration and temporarily reduces your glycogen reserves and the amount of food in your stomach. Dieting therefore starts by psychologically rewarding you for playing scale and mirror games. "My God," you say to yourself, "I've only been on this diet for two days, and already I've lost five pounds! These people sure knew what they were talking about when they told me to eat only mashed yeast and bacon." Then, of course, come those next few depressing days when the scale doesn't show any change at all. "I don't understand," you say to yourself. "I've been so good about eating only mashed yeast and bacon, but I haven't yet lost another five pounds. In fact, I haven't made any progress at all. I guess I'll have to be more patient than I thought." Next comes that awful day when you step on the scale to discover that you've actually regained two pounds! "What's the point of eating nothing but mashed yeast and bacon?" you say to yourself ruefully. "It isn't getting me anywhere in the end. My body has a mind of its own." And there, at last, lies the truth.

But since you are not on a diet, you shouldn't even *want* to know how you are doing each day. You are not on a desperate regime of temporary privation. You will be exercising for the rest of your life. You don't need to see immediate results. Nor will you. You will be gaining muscle at the same time as you are losing fat. Muscle weighs more than fat, so your net weight loss may be relatively small. If you are currently carrying an extra ten pounds of fat, it is possible that you will lose it all while losing only a couple of pounds of measurable net weight. Yet you, and everyone else, will be able to see that your body has been transformed.

Unlike dieting, moreover, your exercise regime is *not* going to cause you to dehydrate or lose your glycogen reserves. You are therefore not going to get that instant reward of five pounds of bulges lost in two days. Don't be disillusioned. Don't stand on the scale looking for it. What's the rush? I assure you that you are going to become and *stay* thin if you keep on exercising, and it's going to happen within a few months. Even within a few weeks, you will notice your body starting to change. What could you hope to accomplish by being alternately elated and depressed by random variations in the water content of your body? All you are doing is increasing the likelihood that you will give up your exercise before you've given it a chance to work.

In any case, you're going to have to learn to trust your body and believe that it really is keeping you thin. You are going to have to stop freaking out because you stepped on the scale the morning after a heavy meal and discovered that you just gained five pounds, even if the mirror appears to confirm the horrible news. You know as a matter of logic that you are being silly. You know that three days from now the extra weight will be gone, and the mirror will confirm that you are still thin. Don't let your fear overpower your logic. Think in a way that is designed to keep you thin in the *long* run.

Have Sensible Goals

Even though you exercise every day, you will eventually reach a point at which you plateau and stop losing fat, because you have reached the new weight that your body wants you to maintain. This will be a slim weight, and everyone will think you look thin and athletic. It will probably be close to the weight that you maintained in your twenties. It is nevertheless possible that there will still be a few ounces of fat on your belly, rear, or waist; that your face may not be as angular as it used to be; that you may not be able to see *all* your ribs; or that you may not have a perfect "washboard stomach." After all, as I explained in chapter 2, healthy, active bodies still maintain some amount of fat as an emergency food store. It is up to your body, not you, to decide how much fat you should have and where to put it. You can't possibly substitute your own judgment for that of your body and maintain your weight in the long run. No matter what you do, moreover, your body will know you are no longer sixteen and looking for a mate. Your body will, in effect, think that it is more important for you to survive and raise the children you already have than it is to make you as angular or curvaceous as you could possibly be.

So before you try to be yet a couple of pounds thinner, I'd like you to stop and consider a few things. First, are you *sure* you would look better even thinner? Maybe you can't be too rich, but you definitely can be too thin. It's easy to lose perspective by focusing on specific parts of your body and on whatever fat deposits they still have. Anorexics always think they look too fat, even just before they die of starvation. Try asking your friends how you look and whether they think you would look better or worse if you were a few pounds thinner. Mirrors can be deceiving. Take some pictures of yourself. Now look at those pictures. That is what you actually look like. Do you really think this person should be thinner?

Second, are you sure the look you are coveting relates to your body fat? A lot of people look their best when they are dehydrated. Dehydration makes your face more angular and your eyes larger. People have been using diuretics as beauty aids for centuries. Dieting initially results in dehydration and therefore offers the dieter an immediate reward, not merely on the scale but in the mirror as well. But the reward is false, because you can't stay dehydrated forever, nor would you want to. Moreover, people notice these minor variations in water bloat less than you realize. Other people are not as focused on the details of your looks as you are. But if it is dehydration you seek, becoming thinner is not going to help you. Your exercise regime is not going to result in dehydration. Neither will any diet, once you go off it. If you want to use diuretics, that's your affair, but don't confuse what you're after with weight loss.

Third, are you sure that having the body of an eighteen-year-old will make you look better to other people? Think about that shapely grandmother you saw on the beach in a pink bikini. Think about that fifty-year-old guy you saw with the open shirt and the chain around his neck, getting out of a red Ferrari. Did you find these people as attractive as they doubtless imagined themselves to be? If not, then what makes you think that if, at age forty, you manage to maintain the body of a teenage supermodel, everyone will think you are an irresistible sex god or goddess? Do you also plan to wear a halter top, a tank top, or a fishnet shirt? Having a teenage body will never make you look like a teenager. Isn't it possible that to sophisticated people, you would look better just being thin? As it says in the Desiderata, "Surrender gracefully the things of youth." You'd better surrender them gracefully, because your only alternative is to surrender them ungracefully, and that can get pretty ugly. People who convey the impression that they are obsessed with their physical appearance also imply that they have little else to offer the world. Is that what you want to communicate to your friends and acquaintances?

But if you really are determined to get rid of *all* of your fat deposits, exercise is not going to help you. Your body will not tolerate leaving you in such a state. It will take the first opportunity to restore the minimum fat deposits it thinks you need to survive the minor variations in food supply that mammals have been encountering since they first stepped out of the seas. People do live with hardly any fat deposits. Some models do, some actors do, and some jockeys do. But they do it by living perpetually on the edge of starvation. They fight their bodies all the time, and they battle each day against the many weapons at their bodies' disposal, from lowered metabolism and depressed mood to food cravings, appetites, and hungers. They are at risk for developing not only physical problems, but also psychological problems of imbalance. In short, they are living relatively unpleasant lives, but at least they are doing it because they *have* to in order to make a living. You don't have to. Why would you want such a life?

Don't Overdo It

We have all experienced the phenomenon of getting excited about something new, whether it be a diet, an exercise regime, a health-food craze, a social approach, or even a form of religious belief. What happens is, first we read something, or hear something, that seems to make sense, and a light goes on. Then we try it, and it seems to succeed. Next, we are zealous converts. It's not enough to just do it. We must *overdo* it. We must talk about it as if it were the focus of our lives. Inevitably, though, we have a relapse. That is no surprise. We could hardly have been expected to maintain such an intensity level. Next we are disillusioned, and we are distracted by other things. Finally, we forget about the whole thing altogether.

The purpose of this book is not to turn you into an exercise nut. I told you in chapter 3 what I think you need to do to stay thin: perform thirty minutes of aerobic exercise every day. I don't want you to do more. I don't want you to exercise for an hour, or two hours, or more each day. The reason is that I don't think you can *sustain* such behavior for the rest of your life. I don't even know why you would want to. It doesn't matter whether even more exercise might help keep you a little bit thinner. Let's start by seeing whether you can sustain any daily regime at all. Let's make a deal. If you have sustained your thirty-minutes-per-day regime for at least one year, then you can consider doing a little more in hopes of being even thinner.

In this regard, I'd like to qualify some advice that I am about to give you. The next chapter talks about weight training. I do think you will store less fat if you can manage to fit in a modest weight-training workout routine twice or three times per week, *in addition to* your aerobic exercise routine. But the aerobic exercise is much more important. Your added muscle will not replace fat if you are basically sedentary. The weight training will be counterproductive if it causes you to devote so much time and effort to exercise that you burn out and stop exercising altogether. No matter how convinced you are right now that this is not going to happen to you, let me assure you that there is a chance that it will. I therefore suggest that you skip over the weightlifting chapter for now and read it if and when you feel sure you have the time and energy to do more on a sustained basis. (But do be sure to read the last chapter on motivation and happiness.)

7.

Low-key Weight Training: Feed a Muscle, Starve a Fat Deposit

AS OLDER PEOPLE BECOME less active and start lifting and stretching less, their bodies need less muscle tissue. They disband the unnecessary tissue, because muscle is expensive to maintain in terms of metabolism—ten times more expensive, in fact, than fat. But the lost muscle tissue was playing an important secondary role: providing their bodies with an emergency food reserve. Their bodies therefore replace the lost reserves with "low-cost" fat deposits. To prevent this from happening, you must persuade your body that it cannot afford to disband your muscle tissue, because you are still hauling foodstuffs, building shelters, carrying children, and so forth. In other words, there is a limit to how much flesh an active person can carry around. If your body takes up most of the available room with muscle, then it will have less room, and less need, for fat.

A modest weight-training routine can serve to persuade your body to maintain its muscle tone and mass. I don't mean, however, that you can opt for weight training *instead* of aerobic exercise. It is possible for sedentary people to carry large amounts of both fat and muscle on their bodies; consider a sumo wrestler. Your muscle is not going to substitute for fat unless your body thinks it must limit its overall bulk, and it will reach that conclusion only if you perform aerobic exercise.

I also don't mean you should have bulging muscles. Your weight training should merely serve to complement your aerobic exercise. Although your aerobic exercise primarily uses the muscles of your lower body, you may also notice an increase in the tone of your upper body as your body reassesses its overall muscular needs in light of its apparently changed life circumstances. After all, someone who is out running after food may also be obliged to carry it home. Your weight training regime serves to confirm your body's assumption that you need more muscle everywhere because you have important and constructive things to do with it.

Your weight training should not take a lot of time. A thirty-minute routine performed two or three times per week should suffice. You don't need to rest for more than fifteen to thirty seconds between sets. By the time you've prepared the next exercise, you should be ready to perform it. Your routine doesn't even have to involve going to the gym. The gym may prove convenient, but you can accomplish everything you need to at home with a simple bench and a few barbells and dumbbells. You can also perform push-ups, sit-ups, and "assisted" pull-ups (as explained below) almost anywhere, whenever you have a moment free and feel in the mood.

In any case, perform ten to twelve different exercises that cover most of your major muscle groups, especially the muscles of your chest, shoulders, and arms (your biceps, triceps, pectoral muscles, and deltoid muscles), since you generally don't use them in your daily exercise. If you do go to a gym, there will probably be a circuit of exercise machines that suits the purpose. You can also work with a trainer there to personalize your routine. If you are using a bench at home, buy a book that takes you through some basic exercise routines.

Whatever you do, don't lift heavy weights or strain your body. Don't try to increase the amount you are lifting over time. Your weight-training workout routine is not a competition, even with yourself, and it is not intended to make you look like a bodybuilder. Your only objectives should be (a) to restore and maintain the muscle tone that you had when you were in your twenties; (b) to do this in a way that takes the minimum amount of time and effort, since life has many other obligations; and (c) to do it without injuring yourself. Straining yourself with heavier weights is completely unnecessary. It won't help you reach your objectives of staying thin and maintaining your muscle tone. All it will do is help you satisfy an illogical (although understandable) desire to feel that you are "getting somewhere" with your weight training. So ignore any well-intended trainers who try to tell you how to "reach your goals" by lifting more weight. Likewise ignore the guys you see at the gym yelling "Push! Push!" at each other for inspiration. Follow instead these three basic rules for weight training:

1. Light weights
2. Slow, controlled lifts
3. Eight to twelve repetitions

Remember that your objective is not really to lift a weight. You are not a construction worker trying to get a job done. Your objective is merely to send a signal to your body that your muscles are not adequate for the task at hand and they therefore need to be built up more (or need to be maintained). This objective does not require you to perform a difficult lift. It only requires you to *continue* lifting until you cannot lift any more—until, in other words, you are forced to stop by your own muscular exhaustion.

This is best accomplished by repeating a relatively easy lift—that is, by doing so-called repetitions. If you are using the proper weight, the first few lifts should be almost effortless. The lifts will gradually become more difficult until you feel the relevant muscles burning as you try to squeeze out another repetition. After a repetition or two in this burn state, the relevant muscles will be exhausted and unable to perform any more repetitions at that weight. It really doesn't matter how much weight you are lifting when this occurs. Your body will get the message as long as it *does* occur. The message is that you would have liked to have lifted more, but you couldn't. You failed to reach your apparent objective. Whatever it was you were trying to accomplish, it must have been important, and your body is going to have to increase the strength of that muscle if you are going to succeed the next time you have to perform.

This objective—lifting to exhaustion—is much easier to achieve with a slow, controlled lift. This means a lift that takes several seconds on the way up, and, just as important, several seconds on the way down, all during which you are in complete control of the placement of the weight. If you could not stop on a dime at any point in the lift and move the weight down again, then you are not in control of the lift. Don't hold your breath. Exhale as you slowly lift the weight up, and breathe in again as you slowly lower it down.

You can, of course, lift more weight with a fast, jerky lift than you can with a slow, controlled one. A fast lift requires your muscles to work against gravity for only a moment, whereas a slow, con-trolled lift forces your muscles to work against gravity for six or seven seconds. Your body will therefore not like performing slow, controlled lifts. "Why are you taking so long to reach your objec-tive?" your body will in effect be asking you on the way up. "This is a lot more work for me. I could get that bar to the top of the arc while expending far less energy." And it will in effect be saying the same thing on the way down. "Why are you taking so long? Why don't you just drop the bar? That will take far less energy." But don't listen to your body. It doesn't understand your objectives. It thinks you are lifting food supplies or shelter materials. The slower you go, the sooner you will reach your burn.

Because a slow, controlled lift requires a lot more energy, you will have to use much lighter weights than you otherwise would. Your first lift should be almost effortless if you are going to remain in perfect control when you reach the burn. Resist the temptation to use too much weight. Otherwise, you will *not* be able to perform a slow, controlled lift when you reach the burn, and you will just wind up kidding yourself about what you are accomplishing.

In other words, when it comes to working out, less is more. Men, please don't feel embarrassed as you take off all those forty-five-pound plates that the other guys in the gym have been using on the bar. They have different objectives and, between you and me, many of them don't have a clue. I promise that you will get *more*, not less, out of your workout if you follow these rules—more muscle and definition for your thirty minutes of effort—than you will if you imitate the people you see around you. And you will continue your workouts long after those people have left the gym to deal, in their thirties and forties, with their bad necks, painful shoulders, aching backs, and pot bellies.

For the most important reason to perform slow, controlled lifts is to avoid injuring yourself. As long as you are performing slow, controlled lifts, you are unlikely to strain or tear your muscles. This is partly because you are not pulling or jerking them. But it is also partly because you have the time and ability to monitor and respond to their signals. In this regard, be sure to listen carefully to your muscles as you perform your repetitions. If any muscle signals the slightest bit of pain, stop the lift immediately and bring the weight slowly back down again. Then stop performing that particular exercise and switch to another muscle group. If the mild pain continues, end the workout session and pick it up again a few days later. You are not doing yourself any favors by pushing onward. One of your muscles has told you that it needs to recover. If you push on, that muscle will be strained, and you will have to stop working out for a week or two. If you make a habit of refusing to listen to your muscles, you may have to stop working out altogether. You must know by now that when it comes to muscle pulls, soft complaints turn out to be much louder the following morning. So listen to your muscles when you're working out.

Be especially careful, in this regard, about your back and neck. Use extralight weights when you are working with them, and be sure you are in total control of any lift. Be careful with sit-ups. Perform them slowly, and don't strain your lower back. Be equally careful with pull-ups. Grasp a *low* overhead bar (or even a thick tree branch), bend your knees, and then use your legs to assist your shoulders and arms with the lift. Apply just enough leg assistance to allow your shoulders and arms to reach a burn after eight repetitions. Don't try to be macho and perform your pull-ups without any leg assistance. Jerky efforts to lift your entire body weight will serve only to injure the muscles of your shoulder and neck.

Finally, note that while it may not matter when the burn develops, it is inefficient to be lifting for too long a period before you develop a burn. You should start with a weight that lets you develop a burn after about eight slow repetitions. Naturally, your muscles will be able to do more repetitions as your strength increases. When you reach the point at which it takes you twelve repetitions to reach a burn, increase the weight by the smallest possible increment.

Also bear in mind that your ability to lift weights will vary from day to day, depending on many factors, such as your blood sugar level, your level of fatigue, and even your mood. Don't worry or be disappointed about using less weight than you generally do. You are not failing, and you are not accomplishing less. Your only objective is to reach your burn. It doesn't matter whether you are doing this with twenty pounds or with thirty. In fact, if you can do it with only twenty, you should be delighted, not disappointed, with your ability to accomplish your desired result so efficiently.

Once you give up competitive lifting, you will be surprised at how easy it is to maintain your muscle tone. It takes relatively little effort to continue having the musculature you had in your early twenties right through your fifties. And unlike competitive lifting, slow, controlled lifting is not unpleasant in the slightest. With competitive lifting, your body realizes that it is in constant danger, and it uses pain and displeasure to try to get you to stop. In effect, your body tries to stop you from pushing it beyond its limits. But with slow, controlled lifting, your body is merely being pushed *to* its limits. It is therefore happy to perform, and it even enjoys the exercise.

8.

Earn Your Daily Happiness

You've probably already noticed that some of the most successful people you know exercise; and, conversely, many of the people you know who exercise are also successful in their lives, both personally and professionally. They have satisfying careers, happy marriages and relationships, and upbeat attitudes that are justified by their fortunate circumstances. You may attribute this to mere coincidence. More likely, you attribute it to correlation. The kinds of people, you think, who have the motivation to exercise also have the motivation to accomplish other important things in their lives. They are those gung-ho people who "do it all." Naturally you see them out jogging at 7:00 a.m. But have you ever considered the possibility that the relation may be partly one of causation? Is it possible that people who perform aerobic exercise are more energetic, more upbeat, more capable, and more motivated, and therefore more successful, *because* they perform aerobic exercise?

When I first learned how to ski, I asked my instructor what I accomplished by planting my pole. "Nothing, really," she told me. "It just lets you tell yourself that you're about to turn yourself around." But, of course, that little nothing is everything. A changed course of human behavior arises from a metaphysical event that occurs within the human mind. Let's call that event a determination to act. Certain determinations to act can have far greater significance, for our lives as a whole, than the immediate actions they produce. In the life of an individual, they can play a role like the one that planting a pole plays in skiing. They can help you turn your whole life around.

The most significant such determination in my own life was when I quit smoking. I was twenty-one, and I had been smoking three packs a day since I was eighteen. I had tried quitting several times before and failed. I had also dropped out of college three times, and I had never held a job for more than two months. One day I told a friend that I was going to stop smoking. Naturally neither my friend nor I expected me to succeed, but in fact I never smoked a cigarette again. Looking back, I realize this was a turning point for me. "If I can say I'm going to quit smoking and then quit," I thought to myself, "then I can say I'm going to finish college and finish it." And indeed after that, finishing college turned out to be easy.

Taking control of your life, accomplishing objectives, conducting your affairs with energy and interest, these are all human actions that arise out of inner determinations. For people who are not in the daily habit of motivating themselves, these actions can seem very difficult. Such people are motivationally out of shape. But all motivation is fundamentally the same. The motivation to perform physical tasks does not differ in substance from the motivation to perform psychological ones. You get used to performing both if you are in the habit of performing, and if you are in the habit of performing, it's easy to perform.

Of course it seems unpleasant at first to perform thirty minutes per day of aerobic exercise. But you *can* determine to do it and stick to it. The amazing part is not that you actually can, but rather that if you do, it stops being difficult and unpleasant and becomes relatively easy. In part, this is because your body gets in shape, and has fewer problems physically performing the exercise. But the more important reason is that your *mind* gets in shape and stops complaining about the exercise. You even start to look forward to the exercise. You find yourself enjoying the opportunity to drive your body's muscles forward and to feel their health, their energy, and their youth. And if you stick to it, you will realize in a few months that you have gone from being a person who is habitually inert to one who is habitually active. You will find, in other words, that you have changed fundamentally as a person.

If you can go from being someone who is sedentary, who is physically passive, and who is therefore chubby or flabby, to being someone who is intentionally active, who is physically controlled, and who is therefore thin and toned, and if you can *sustain* that change and make it permanent, then you are sure to find it easier to take the next step. If you have been habitually passive in your career, you will find it easier to get up early and write the necessary articles, papers, presentations, books, memos, analyses, and so forth that will take your career to the next level. If you have been habitually passive in social interactions, you will find it easier to focus on other people, to remember their names, objectives, and interests, and to adapt and respond to their facial expressions and actions. If you have been habitually passive in personal relationships, you will find it easier to focus energetically on your spouse or companion, children, friends, and family relations and radiate a positive energy and attitude.

None of these changes is easy. All of them take time. All of them are gradual processes of reinvention. But all of them are possible, and all of them are well within your grasp. The one thing they require is determination, *daily* determination. If you succeed in performing thirty minutes of aerobic exercise each day, it will be easier for you to find that determination, and make those changes, for two reasons. First, you will have more energy. Your exercise will give you the lift you need to feel energetic for the entire day.

Second, and more important, you will already be in the habit of commanding and controlling yourself. You will already be in the habit of telling yourself what to do. And the parts of yourself that need to listen and change will already be in the habit of listening and changing. They will already be in the habit of taking orders from the highest part of your brain.

Dieting will not help you accomplish these things. Dieting is not an exercise in self-control, as most people think. Dieting is an exercise in self-*denial*. Dieting does not involve driving the will forward. It involves holding it back. The person who gets in the habit of self-denial soon moves on to denying others. Dieting deprives your body and your mind of energy. Dieting therefore leads to sluggish, depressed, and unbalanced behavior. Exercise, on the other hand, harnesses your body's resources to produce and radiate energy. There is therefore an enormous difference in the respective shadows that dieting and exercise cast over your life. Dieting leads you to stop doing; exercise leads you to start doing. Dieting leads you to do less; exercise leads you to do more. Dieting leads you to back off; exercise leads you to forge ahead. Dieting leads you to lie down; exercise leads you to stand up.

None of us can know *why* there is life. But all of us know what life *is*. Life is an active biological force that moves in a direction opposite to the physical forces of entropy and inertia. Entropy and inertia wear things down, and apart from life, they govern the universe. Apart from life, things degenerate, decay, and otherwise move toward a state of randomness. Yet in the very face of such forces life maintains, builds up, creates, produces, and extends. Life is the force that continually sweeps the dust out of the house that the wind keeps blowing in. It is the force that takes two steps forward after being pushed one step back; that raises up generations, even when some of them are lost; that builds houses and businesses and skyscrapers; that develops new bodies of knowledge and new technologies. Life is the force of energy, energy that comes from within. None of us can say whether the energy is justified, but none of us can deny that life is about radiating it.

When we die, we will lie down and decay, and we will perform no more. Some may be ready to start right now, and who is to say they are wrong? Some may not be sure they want to give up just yet, so they have decided to give up halfway by doing as little as possible. But for the rest of us, who want to embrace life, life is about energy. Life is about doing and accomplishing and taking on challenges. And the funny thing about life's accomplishments is, they never seem easy at first. They always feel like a bit of a push. But after you get over the initial hump, they always feel wonderful, because that is all life has to offer, that is all life is.

If you think you would be happier doing nothing constructive, then you are wrong about yourself. Life is about accomplishment, and you will lose your happiness the moment you stop accomplishing, just as you will lose your thinness the moment you stop exercising. What makes people happy is not what they are, or what they have, but what they *do*! That means you have to create your own happiness every day, no matter how successful you were yesterday. Doing thirty minutes per day of aerobic exercise will not *ensure* your daily happiness, but it will start you out in the right direction.

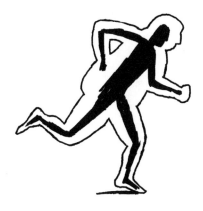

Acknowledgments

My sincere thanks to:

Judith Appelbaum (and Sensible Solutions), without whom this book would not have been possible;
Tod Lippy, for his careful reading and advice;
Jennifer Sisk, for her excellent research;
Scott Menchin, for his smart illustrations;
Judith Stein, for her thorough copyediting;
Richard Dawkins, for writing *The Selfish Gene;*
and the staff of Cypress House, for all their hard work.

Bibliography

Chapter 1
Is Your Body Really Just a Passive Fat Depository?

Allen, John S., and Susan M. Cheer. "The Non-thrifty Genotype." *Current Anthropology* 37 (December 1996): 831–42.

Baile, C. A., M. A. Della-Fera, and R. J. Martin. "Regulation of Metabolism and Body Fat Mass by Leptin." *Annual Review of Nutrition* 20 (2000): 105–27.

Bulik, C. M., and D. B. Allison. "The Genetic Epidemiology of Thinness." *Obesity Reviews* 2, no. 2 (May 2001): 107–15.

Cannon, Joseph P. G. "The Hunger Hormone." *Today's Dietitian* (February 2003): 44–45.

Centers for Disease Control and Prevention. "Physical Activity Trends—United States, 1990–1998." *Journal of the American Medical Association* 285, no. 14 (April 11, 2001): 1835.

Doucet, E., et al. "Appetite After Weight Loss by Energy Restriction and a Low-fat Diet-Exercise Follow-up." *International Journal of Obesity and Related Metabolic Disorders* 24, no. 7 (July 2000): 906–14.

Figueroa-Colon, R., et al. "Paternal Body Fat Is a Longitudinal Predictor of Changes in Body Fat in Premenarcheal Girls." *American Journal of Clinical Nutrition* 71, no. 3 (March 2000): 829–34.

Flegal, K. M., et al. "Prevalence and Trends in Obesity Among U.S. Adults, 1999–2000." *Journal of the American Medical Association* 288, no. 14 (October 9, 2002): 1723–7.

Havel, P. J. "Role of Adipose Tissue in Body-Weight Regulation:

Mechanisms Regulating Leptin Production and Energy Balance." *Proceedings of the Nutrition Society* 59, no. 3 (August 2000): 359–71.

Heitmann, B. L., et al. "Genetic Effects on Weight Change and Food Intake in Swedish Adult Twins." *American Journal of Clinical Nutrition* 69, no. 4 (April 1999): 597–602.

Kahn, J. "Exercise and Not Genetics Is Major Determinant of Weight, Study Finds." May 16, 1996. Ernest Orlando Lawrence Berkeley National Laboratory. <http://www.lbl.gov/Science-Articles/Archive/exercise-weight.html> (Last accessed July 28, 2003.)

Korkeila, M., et al. "Weight-loss Attempts and Risk of Major Weight Gain: A Prospective Study in Finnish Adults." *American Journal of Clinical Nutrition* 70, no. 6 (December 1999): 965–75.

Norgan, N. G. "The Beneficial Effects of Body Fat and Adipose Tissue in Humans." *International Journal of Obesity and Related Metabolic Disorders* 21, no. 9 (September 1997): 738–46.

Ogden, C. L., et al. "Prevalence and Trends in Overweight Among U.S. Children and Adolescents, 1999–2000." *Journal of the American Medical Association* 288, no. 14 (October 9, 2002): 1728–32.

Peters, J. C., et al. "From Instinct to Intellect: the Challenge of Maintaining Healthy Weight in the Modern World." *Obesity Reviews* 3, no. 2 (May 2002): 69–74.

Plowman, Sharon A., and Denise L. Smith. *Exercise Physiology for Health, Fitness, and Performance.* 2nd ed. New York: Benjamin Cummings, 2003.

Rao, D. C., and C. Bouchard. "Familial Aggregation of Amount and Distribution of Subcutaneous Fat and Their Responses to Exercise Training in the HERITAGE Family Study." *Obesity Research* 8, no. 2 (March 2000): 140–50.

Samaras, K., et al. "Genetic and Environmental Influences on Total-body and Central Abdominal Fat: The Effect of Physical Activity in Female Twins." *Annals of Internal Medicine* 130, no. 11 (June 1, 1999): 873–82.

Samaras, K., et al. "Independent Genetic Factors Determine the Amount and Distribution of Fat in Women After the Menopause." *Journal of Clinical Endocrinology and Metabolism* 82, no. 3 (March 1997): 781–5.

Serdula, M. K., et al. "Prevalence of Attempting Weight Loss and Strategies for Controlling Weight." *Journal of the American Medical Association* 282, no. 14 (October 13, 1999): 1353–8.

Stunkard, A. J., et al. "Energy Intake, Not Energy Output, Is a Determinant of Body Size in Infants." *American Journal of Clinical Nutrition* 69, no. 3 (March 1999): 524–30.

Thorburn, A. W., and J. Proietto. "Biological Determinants of Spontaneous Physical Activity." *Obesity Reviews* 1, no. 2 (October 2000): 87–94.

Weinsier, R. L., et al. "The Etiology of Obesity: Relative Contribution of Metabolic Factors, Diet, and Physical Activity." *American Journal of Medicine* 105, no. 2 (August 1998): 145–50.

Weinsier, R. L. "Genes and Obesity: Is There Reason to Change Our Behaviors?" *Annals of Internal Medicine* 130, no. 11 (June 1, 1999): 938–9.

Chapter 2
Storing Fat Was a Bad Evolutionary Strategy— Except in One Case

Chen, J. D. "Evolutionary Aspects of Exercise." *World Review of Nutrition and Dietetics* 84 (1999): 106–17.

Brozek, Josef. "Quantitative Description of Body Composition: Physical Anthropology's 'Fourth' Dimension." *Current Anthropology* 4 (February 1963): 3–39.

Carrier, David R. "The Energetic Paradox of Human Running and Hominid Evolution." *Current Anthropology* 25, no. 4 (August–October 1984): 483–95.

Cordain, L., et al. "Physical Activity, Energy Expenditure and Fitness: An Evolutionary Perspective." *International Journal of Sports Medicine* 19, no. 5 (July 1998): 328–35.

Cordain, L., R. W. Gotshall, and S. B. Eaton. "Evolutionary Aspects of Exercise." *World Review of Nutrition and Dietetics* 81 (1997): 49–60.

Dufour, D. L., and M. L. Sauther. "Comparative and Evolutionary Dimensions of the Energetics of Human Pregnancy and Lactation." *American Journal of Human Biology* 14, no. 5 (September–October 2002): 584–602.

Friedrich, M. J. "Epidemic of Obesity Expands Its Spread to Developing Countries." *Journal of the American Medical Association* 287, no. 11 (March 20, 2002): 1382–6.

Hawkes, K., J. F. O'Connell, and N. G. Blurton Jones. "Hadza Women's Time Allocation, Offspring Provisioning, and the Evolution of Long Postmenopausal Life Spans." *Current Anthropology* 38 (August–October, 1997): 551–77.

Hawkes, K., J. F. O'Connell, and N. G. Blurton Jones. "Hunting and Nuclear Families." *Current Anthropology* 42 (2001): 681–709.

Johnson, Rachel K. "Changing Eating and Physical Activity Patterns of U.S. Children." *Proceedings of the Nutrition Society* 59 (2000): 295–301.

Kassirer, J. P., and M. Angell. "Losing Weight: An Ill-fated New Year's Resolution." *New England Journal of Medicine* 338, no. 1 (January 1998):52–4.

Leibel, R. L., M. Rosenbaum, and J. Hirsch. "Changes in Energy Expenditure Resulting from Altered Body Weight." *New England Journal of Medicine* 332, no. 10 (March 1995): 621–8.

LeMura, L. M., and M. T. Maziekas. "Factors That Alter Body Fat, Body Mass, and Fat-free Mass in Pediatric Obesity." *Medicine and Science in Sports and Exercise* 34, no. 3 (March 2002): 487–96.

MacDonald, Douglas H., and Barry S. Hewlett. "Reproductive Interests and Forager Mobility." *Current Anthropology* 40 (August–October 1999): 501–23.

Marlowe, F. "Male Contribution to Diet and Female Reproductive Success Among Foragers." *Current Anthropology* 42, no. 5 (December 2001): 755–9.

O'Connell, J. F., K. Hawkes, and N. G. Blurton Jones. "Hadza Scavenging: Implications for Plio/Pleistocene Hominid Subsistence." *Current Anthropology* 29, no. 2 (April 1988): 356–63.

O'Connell, J. F., K. Hawkes, and N. G. Blurton Jones. "Grandmothering and the Evolution of *Homo erectus*." *Journal of Human Evolution* 36, no. 5 (May 1999): 461–85.

Panter-Brick, C. "Sexual Division of Labor: Energetic and Evolutionary Scenarios." *American Journal of Human Biology* 14, no. 5 (September–October 2002): 627–40.

Pawlowski, Boguslaw. "The Evolution of Gluteal/Femoral Fat Deposits and Balance During Pregnancy in Bipedal *Homo*." *Current Anthropology* 42, no. 4 (August–October 2001): 572–4.

Peccei, J. S. "A Critique of the Grandmother Hypotheses: Old and New." *American Journal of Human Biology* 13, no. 4 (July–August 2001): 434–52.

Peccei, J. S. "A Hypothesis for the Origin and Evolution of Menopause." *Maturitas* 21, no. 2 (February 1995): 83–9.

Peccei, J. S. "First Estimates of Heritability in the Age of Menopause." *Current Anthropology* 40 (August–October 1999): 553–8.

Perusse, L., et al. "Familial Aggregation of Amount and Distribution of Subcutaneous Fat and Their Responses to Exercise Training in the HERITAGE Family Study." *Obesity Research* 8, no. 2 (March 2000): 140–50.

Pond, C. M. "The Biological Origins of Adipose Tissue." In *The Evolving Female: A Life History Perspective*, edited by Mary Ellen Morbeck, Alison Galloway, and Adrienne L. Zihlman. E-book edition. Princeton, N.J.: Princeton University Press, 2001, 147–62.

Rose, Lisa, and Fiona Marshall. "Meat Eating, Hominid Sociality, and Home Bases Revisited." *Current Anthropology* 37 (April 1996): 307–38.

Sherman, P. W. "The Evolution of Menopause." *Nature* 392 (April 23, 1998): 759.

Sorensen, M. V., and W. R. Leonard. "Neandertal Energetics and Foraging Efficiency." *Journal of Human Evolution* 40, no. 6 (June 2001): 483–95.

Stanford, C.B., and H. T. Bunn. 1999. "Meat Eating and Hominid Evolution." *Current Anthropology* 40, no. 5 (December 1999): 726–8.

Strassmann, Beverly I. "The Biology of Menstruation in *Homo sapiens*: Total Lifetime Menses, Fecundity, and Nonsynchrony in a Natural-fertility Population." *Current Anthropology* 38 (February 1997): 123–9.

Sykes, Bryan. *The Seven Daughters of Eve*. New York: W. W. Norton and Company, 2001.

Testart, A. "The Significance of Food Storage Among Hunter-Gatherers: Residence Patterns, Population Densities, and Social Inequalities." *Current Anthropology* 23, no. 5 (October 1982): 523–37.

Thorburn, A. W., and J. Proietto. "Biological Determinants of Spontaneous Physical Activity." *Obesity Reviews* 1, no. 2 (October 2000):87–94.

Treuth, M. S., et al. "Familial Resemblance of Body Composition in Prepubertal Girls and Their Biological Parents." *American Journal of Clinical Nutrition* 74, no. 4 (October 2001): 529–33.

Walker, A. R., B. F. Walker, and F. Adam. "Nutrition, Diet, Physical Activity, Smoking, and Longevity: From Primitive Hunter-Gatherer to Present Passive Consumer—How Far Can We Go?" *Nutrition* 19, no. 2 (February 2003): 169–73.

Chapter 3
How to Make Your Body Think You Run for a Living

American College of Sports Medicine Position Stand. "The Recommended Quantity and Quality of Exercise for Developing and Maintaining Cardiorespiratory and Muscular Fitness and Flexibility in Healthy Adults." *Medicine and Science in Sports and Exercise* 30, no. 6 (June 1998): 975–91.

Andersen, R. E., et al. "Effects of Lifestyle Activity Vs. Structured Aerobic Exercise in Obese Women: A Randomized Trial." *Journal of the American Medical Association* 281, no. 4 (January 27, 1999): 335–40.

Andersen, R. E., et al. "Physiologic Changes After Diet Combined with Structured Aerobic Exercise or Lifestyle Activity." *Metabolism* 51, no. 12 (December 2002): 1528–33.

Berle, A. Lynn. *Water Aerobics*. 2nd ed. Dubuque, Iowa: Kendall/Hunt Publishing, 1996.

Bond, Brill J., et al. "Dose-Response Effect of Walking Exercise on Weight Loss: How Much Is Enough?" *International Journal of Obesity and Related Metabolic Disorders* 26, no. 11 (November 2002): 1484–93.

Burke, Edmund R. *Precision Heartrate Training*. 2nd ed. Champaign, Ill.: Human Kinetics, 1998.

Dionne, I, et al. "The Association Between Vigorous Physical Activities and Fat Deposition in Male Adolescents." *Medicine and Science in Sports and Exercise* 32, no. 2 (February 2000): 392–5.

DiPietro, L., et al. "Improvements in Cardiorespiratory Fitness Attenuate Age-related Weight Gain in Healthy Men and Women: The Aerobics Center Longitudinal Study." *International Journal of Obesity and Related Metabolic Disorders* 22, no. 1 (January 1998): 55–62.

Dunn, A. L., et al. "Comparison of Lifestyle and Structured Interventions to Increase Physical Activity and Cardiorespiratory Fitness: A Randomized Trial." *Journal of the American Medical Association* 281, no. 4 (January 27, 1999): 327–34.

Erlichman, J., A. L. Kerbey, and W. P. James. "Physical Activity and Its Impact on Health Outcomes. 1. The Impact of Physical Activity on Cardiovascular Disease and All-cause Mortality: An Historical Perspective." *Obesity Reviews* 3, no. 4 (November 2002): 257–71.

Erlichman, J., A. L. Kerbey, and W. P. James. "Physical Activity and Its Impact on Health Outcomes. 2. Prevention of Unhealthy Weight Gain and Obesity by Physical Activity: An Analysis of the Evidence." *Obesity Reviews* 3, no. 4 (November 2002): 273–87.

Fogelholm, M, and K. Kukkonen-Harjula. "Does Physical Activity Prevent Weight Gain? A Systematic Review." *Obesity Reviews* 1, no. 2 (October 2000): 95–111.

Hill, J. O., and R. Commerford. "Physical Activity, Fat Balance, and Energy Balance." *International Journal of Sport Nutrition* 6, no. 2 (June 1996): 80–92.

Hunter, G. R., et al. "A Role for High Intensity Exercise on Energy Balance and Weight Control." *International Journal of Obesity and Related Metabolic Disorders* 22, no. 6 (June 1998): 489–93.

Iknoian, Therese. *Walking Fast*. Champaign, Ill.: Human Kinetics, 1998.

Institute of Medicine. "Dietary Reference Intakes for Energy, Carbohydrate, Fiber, Fat, Fatty Acids, Cholesterol, Protein, and Amino Acids." September 2002. Available free on the Web at <http://www.nap.edu/books/0309085373/html>.

Irwin, M. L., et al. "Effect of Exercise on Total and Intra-abdominal Body Fat in Postmenopausal Women: A Randomized Controlled Trial." *Journal of the American Medical Association* 289, no. 3 (January 15, 2003): 323–30.

Jakicic, J. M. "The Role of Physical Activity in Prevention and Treatment of Body Weight Gain in Adults." *Journal of Nutrition* 132, no. 12 (December 2002): 3826S–9S.

Jakicic, J. M., et al. "Effects of Intermittent Exercise and Use of Home Exercise Equipment on Adherence, Weight Loss, and Fitness in Overweight Women: A Randomized Trial." *Journal of the American Medical Association* 282, no. 16 (October 27, 1999): 1554–60.

Jakicic, J. M., et al. American College of Sports Medicine position stand. "Appropriate Intervention Strategies for Weight Loss and Prevention of Weight Regain for Adults." *Medicine and Science in Sports and Exercise* 33, no. 12 (December 2001): 2145–56.

Jakicic, J. M., et al. "Effect of exercise duration and intensity on weight loss in overweight, sedentary women: A randomized trial." *Journal of the American Medical Association* 290, no. 10 (September 10, 2003): 1323–30.

Klausen, B., et al. "Increased Intensity of a Single Exercise Bout Stimulates Subsequent Fat Intake." *International Journal of Obesity and Related Metabolic Disorders* 23, no. 12 (December 1999): 1282–7.

Kriketos, A. D., et al. "Effects of Aerobic Fitness on Fat Oxidation and Body Fatness." *Medicine and Science in Sports and Exercise* 32, no. 4 (April 2000): 805–11.

Laird, Ron. *Fast Walking*. Mechanicsburg, Pa.: Stackpole Books, 2000.

Mayo, M. J., J. R. Grantham, and G. Balasekaran. "Exercise-induced Weight Loss Preferentially Reduces Abdominal Fat." *Medicine and Science in Sports and Exercise* 35, no. 2 (February 2003): 207–13.

Miller W. C., D. M. Koceja, and E. J. Hamilton. "A Meta-analysis of the

Past 25 Years of Weight Loss Research Using Diet, Exercise or Diet Plus Exercise Intervention." *International Journal of Obesity and Related Metabolic Disorders* 21, no. 10 (October 1997): 941–7.

Parizkova, Jana. "Body Composition and Physical Fitness." *Current Anthropology* 9 (October 1968): 273–87.

Plowman, Sharon A., and Denise L. Smith. *Exercise Physiology for Health, Fitness, and Performance.* 2nd ed. New York: Benjamin Cummings, 2003.

Pryor, Esther, and Minda Goodman Kraines. *Keep Moving! Fitness Through Aerobics and Step.* 4th ed. New York: McGraw-Hill, 1999.

Riddoch, Chris, and Jim McKenna, eds. *Perspectives on Health and Exercise.* London: Macmillan, 2003.

Schmidt, W. D., C. J. Biwer, and L. K. Kalscheuer. "Effects of Long Versus Short Bout Exercise on Fitness and Weight Loss in Overweight Females." *Journal of the American College of Nutrition* 20, no. 5 (October 2001): 494–501.

Sherwood, N. E., et al. "Predictors of Weight Gain in the Pound of Prevention Study." *International Journal of Obesity and Related Metabolic Disorders* 24, no. 4 (April 2000): 395–403.

Smith, D. A., et al. "Resting Metabolic Rate, Body Composition and Aerobic Fitness Comparisons Between Active and Sedentary 54–71 Year Old Males." *European Journal of Clinical Nutrition* 53, no. 6 (June 1999): 434–40.

Snyder, K. A., et al. "The Effects of Long-term, Moderate Intensity, Intermittent Exercise on Aerobic Capacity, Body Composition, Blood Lipids, Insulin and Glucose in Overweight Females." *International Journal of Obesity and Related Metabolic Disorders* 21, no. 12 (December 1997): 1180–9.

Takeshima, N., et al. "Water-based Exercise Improves Health-related Aspects of Fitness in Older Women." *Medicine and Science in Sports and Exercise* 34, no. 3 (March 2002): 544–51.

Thomas, E. L., et al. "Preferential Loss of Visceral Fat Following Aerobic Exercise, Measured by Magnetic Resonance Imaging." *Lipids* 35, no. 7 (July 2000): 769–76.

van Aggel-Leijssen, D. P., et al. "The Effect of Low-intensity Exercise Training on Fat Metabolism of Obese Women." *Obesity Research* 9, no. 2 (February 2001): 86–96.

Votruba, S. B., et al. "Prior Exercise Increases Subsequent Utilization of Dietary Fat." *Medicine and Science in Sports and Exercise* 34, no. 11 (November 2002): 1757–65.

Wagner, A., et al. ""Leisure-time Physical Activity and Regular Walking or Cycling to Work Are Associated with Adiposity and 5 Y Weight Gain in Middle-aged Men: The PRIME Study." *International Journal of Obesity and Related Metabolic Disorders* 25, no. 7 (July 2001): 940–8.

Weinsier, R. L., et al. "Free-living Activity Energy Expenditure in Women Successful and Unsuccessful at Maintaining a Normal Body Weight." *American Journal of Clinical Nutrition* 75, no. 3 (March 2002): 499–504.

Westerterp, K. R., and M. I. Goran. "Relationship Between Physical Activity Related Energy Expenditure and Body Composition: A Gender Difference." *International Journal of Obesity and Related Metabolic Disorders* 21, no. 3 (March 1997): 184–8.

Wier, L. T., et al. "Determining the Amount of Physical Activity Needed for Long-term Weight Control." *International Journal of Obesity and Related Metabolic Disorders* 25, no. 5 (May 2001): 613–21.

World Health Organization. "Diet, Nutrition and the Prevention of Chronic Diseases." World Health Organization Technical Report Service 916, nos. i–viii (2003): 1–149.

Yoshioka, M., et al. "Impact of High-intensity Exercise on Energy Expenditure, Lipid Oxidation and Body Fatness." *International Journal of Obesity and Related Metabolic Disorders* 25, no. 3 (March 2001): 332–9.

Chapter 4
Jack Sprat Was on Pritikin, His Wife Was on Atkins

Brown, R. C., C. M. Cox, and A. Goulding. "High-carbohydrate Versus High-fat Diets: Effect on Body Composition in Trained Cyclists." *Medicine and Science in Sports and Exercise* 32, no. 3 (March 2000): 690–4.

Cheuvront, S. N. "The Zone Diet Phenomenon: A Closer Look at the Science Behind the Claims." *Journal of the American College of Nutrition* 22, no. 1 (February 2003): 9–17.

Chin-Chance, C., K. S. Polonsky, and D. A. Schoeller. "Twenty-four-hour Leptin Levels Respond to Cumulative Short-term Energy Imbalance and Predict Subsequent Intake." *Journal of Clinical Endocrinology and Metabolism* 85, no. 8 (August 2000): 2685–91.

Chu, N. F., et al. "Dietary and Lifestyle Factors in Relation to Plasma Leptin Concentrations Among Normal Weight and Overweight Men." *International Journal of Obesity and Related Metabolic Disorders* 25, no. 1 (January 2001): 106–14.

Dirks, Robert. "Social Responses During Severe Food Shortages and Famine." *Current Anthropology* 21, no. 1 (February 1980): 21–44.

Eisenstein, J., et al. "High-protein Weight-loss Diets: Are They Safe and Do They Work? A Review of the Experimental and Epidemiologic Data." *Nutrition Review* 60, no. 7, part 1 (July 2002): 189–200.

Gingras, J. R., et al. "Metabolic Assessment of Female Chronic Dieters with Either Normal or Low Resting Energy Expenditures." *American Journal of Clinical Nutrition* 71, no. 6 (June 2000): 1413–20.

Larkin, M. "Little Agreement About How to Slim Down the USA." *Lancet* 360 (November 2002): 1400.

Moore, M. S. "Interactions Between Physical Activity and Diet in the Regulation of Body Weight." *Proceedings of the Nutrition Society* 59, no. 2 (May 2000): 193–8.

Nindl, B. C., et al. "Leptin Concentrations Experience a Delayed Reduction After Resistance Exercise in Men." *Medicine and Science in Sports and Exercise* 34, no. 4 (April 2002): 608–13.

Shiiya, T., et al. "Plasma Ghrelin Levels in Lean and Obese Humans and the Effect of Glucose on Ghrelin Secretion." *Journal of Clinical Endocrinology and Metabolism* 87, no. 1 (January 2002): 240–4.

Visona, C., and V. A. George. "Impact of Dieting Status and Dietary Restraint on Postexercise Energy Intake in Overweight Women." *Obesity Research* 10, no. 12 (December 2002): 1251–8.

Willett, W. C., and R. L. Leibel. "Dietary Fat Is Not a Major Determinant of Body Fat." *American Journal of Medicine* 113, supplement 9B (December 2002): 47S–59S.

Wrangham, R. W., et al. "The Raw and the Stolen: Cooking and Human Origins." *Current Anthropology* 40 (December 1999): 567–94.

Wren, A. M., et al. "Ghrelin Enhances Appetite and Increases Food Intake in Humans." *Journal of Clinical Endocrinology and Metabolism* 86, no. 12 (December 2001): 5992.

Chapter 5
Eat When You're Hungry, Stop When You're Full

Anderson, J. W., et al. "Long-term Weight-loss Maintenance: A Meta-analysis of U.S. Studies." *American Journal of Clinical Nutrition* 74, no. 5 (November 2001): 579–84.

Bennett, W. I. "Beyond Overeating." *New England Journal of Medicine* 332, no. 10 (March 1995): 673–4.

Brodney, S., et al. "Nutrient Intake of Physically Fit and Unfit Men and Women." *Medicine and Science in Sports and Exercise* 33, no. 3 (March 2001): 459–67.

Cordain, L., et al. "Influence of Moderate Daily Wine Consumption on Body Weight Regulation and Metabolism in Healthy Free-living Males." *Journal of the American College of Nutrition* 16, no. 2 (April 1997): 134–9.

Critser, G. *Fat Land: How Americans Became the Fattest People in the World.* Boston: Houghton Mifflin, 2003.

Cummings, S., E. S. Parham, and G. W. Strain. "Position of the American Dietetic Association: Weight Management." *Journal of the American Dietetic Association* 102, no. 8 (August 2002): 1145–55.

Drummond, S. E., et al. "Evidence That Eating Frequency Is Inversely Related to Body Weight Status in Male, but Not Female, Non-obese Adults Reporting Valid Dietary Intakes." *International Journal of Obesity and Related Metabolic Disorders* 22, no. 2 (February 1998): 105–12.

King, N. A. "What Processes Are Involved in the Appetite Response to Moderate Increases in Exercise-induced Energy Expenditure?" *Proceedings of the Nutrition Society* 58, no. 1 (February 1999): 107–13.

Schutz, Y. "The Adjustment of Energy Expenditure and Oxidation to Energy Intake: The Role of Carbohydrate and Fat Balance." *International Journal of Obesity and Related Metabolic Disorders* 17, supplement 3 (December 1993): S23–7; discussion S41–2.

Simon, Harvey B. "Diet and Exercise." August 2001. WebMD *Scientific American Medicine*. Available on the Web by subscription at <http://www.samed.com>

Zhang, J., E. H. Temme, and H. Kesteloot. "Alcohol Drinkers Overreport Their Energy Intake in the Birnh Study: Evaluation by 24–Hour Urinary Excretion of Cations." Belgian Interuniversity Research on Nutrition and Health. *Journal of the American College of Nutrition* 20, no. 5 (October 2001): 510–9.

Chapter 6
Stop Obsessing About Your Weight

Abraham, S. "Eating and Weight Controlling Behaviours of Young Ballet Dancers." *Psychopathology* 29, no. 4 (1996): 218–22.

Burley, V.J., et al. "Across-the-Day Monitoring

of Mood And Energy Intake Before, During, and After a Very-Low-Calorie Diet." *American Journal of Clinical Nutrition* 56, supplement 1 (July 1992): 277S–8S.

Kreitzman, S. N., A. Y. Coxon, and K. F. Szaz. "Glycogen Storage: Illusions of Easy Weight Loss, Excessive Weight Regain, and Distortions in Estimates of Body Composition." *American Journal of Clinical Nutrition* 56, supplement 1 (July 1992): 292S–3S.

Oppliger, R. A., S.A. Steen, and J. R. Scott. "Weight Loss Practices of College Wrestlers." *International Journal of Sport Nutrition and Exercise Metabolism* 13, no. 1 (March 2003): 29–46.

Plowman, Sharon A., and Denise L. Smith. *Exercise Physiology for Health, Fitness, and Performance.* 2nd ed. New York: Benjamin Cummings, 2003.

Chapter 7
Low-key Weight Training: Feed a Muscle, Starve a Fat Deposit

Ahmed, C., W. Hilton, and K. Pituch. "Relations of Strength Training to Body Image Among a Sample of Female University Students." *Journal of Strength and Conditioning Research* 16, no. 4 (November 2002): 645–8.

Baechle, T.R., and R. W. Earle, eds. *Essentials of Strength Training and Conditioning.* 2nd ed. Champaign, Ill.: Human Kinetics, 2000.

Borg, P., et al. "Effects of Walking or Resistance Training on Weight Loss Maintenance in Obese, Middle-aged Men: A Randomized Trial." *International Journal of Obesity and Related Metabolic Disorders* 26, no. 5 (May 2002): 676–83.

Hunter, G. R., et al. "Resistance Training and Intra-abdominal Adipose Tissue in Older Men and Women." *Medicine and Science in Sports and Exercise* 34, no. 6 (June 2002): 1023–8.

Kraemer, W. J., et al. American College of Sports Medicine position stand. "Progression Models in Resistance Training for Healthy Adults." *Medicine and Science in Sports and Exercise* 34, no. 2 (February 2002): 364–80.

Plowman, Sharon A., and Denise L. Smith. *Exercise Physiology for Health, Fitness, and Performance.* 2nd ed. New York: Benjamin Cummings, 2003.

Pollock, M. L., et al. AHA Science Advisory. "Resistance Exercise in Individuals with and Without Cardiovascular Disease: Benefits, Rationale, Safety, and Prescription." An Advisory from the Committee on Exercise, Rehabilitation, and Prevention, Council on Clinical Cardiology, American Heart Association. Position paper endorsed by the American College of Sports Medicine. *Circulation* 101, no. 7 (February 22, 2000): 828–33.

Index

Exercise
Frustration, 1, 34, 63

G

Genetics. *See also* Evolution
   "active, thin/sedentary, fat"
      gene, 13-15, 19-20, 22, 25
Goals, 79-81
Gym, 35, 44, 84. *See also* Exercise

H

Heart, 17, 29, 30, 34, 38. *See also*
   Heart rate
Heart rate. *See also* Exercise
   levels of during exercise, 28
      cardiac drift, 33
      charts for, 34
      jogging, 37-38, 39
      Karvonen method, 32
      monitoring, 30-33
      resting heart rate, 31
      target heart rate, 31-32, 34,
         43, 46-47
Hunger. *See also* Appetite; Eating
   adult hunger, 72-73
   natural patterns for, 67, 71-72
   relation to eating, 57-58, 71-72

I

Illness, 18
   exercise and, 25, 51
   fat storage and, 13-14, 18-19
   obesity as, 63-64
   risk of, 30, 81
Injury, 18, 38, 44
   fat storage and, 13-14, 18-19
   weight training, 85, 87-88

J

Jogging, 27-28, 50. *See also*
   Exercise; Running
   aqua-jogging, 43-44
   compared to fast walking, 37,
      42
   do's and don'ts for, 37-41
   heart rate and, 37-38, 39
   indoors, 43
   marathons, 29, 40-41
   not a competitive activity, 38,
      40
   outdoor jogging, 37-41, 49
   physical impacts of, 36, 37, 39,
      41
   on treadmill, 36

K

Karvonen method, 32

L

Lamarck, Jean-Baptiste de Monet
   de, 11, 12, 52
Leptin, 7, 58, 72
Life force, 94-95
Lifestyle
   exercise as part of, 28-29, 93
   interplay with genetics, 11-12
   mealtimes, 71-72
   sedentary lifestyle effects, 8-9,
      13-26, 40, 57-58, 65, 83-84
Lipostat, 6-7. *See also* Body

M

Meaning of Life, The, 67-68
Metabolism. *See also* Body
   factors affecting, 7
Mind. *See also* Attitude